GREAT EXPECTATIONS
TWENTY-FIVE TRUE STORIES
ABOUT CHILDBIRTH

Edited by
Dede Crane and Lisa Moore

First published in Canada in 2008 and the USA in 2008 by House of Anansi Press Inc.
This edition published in Canada in 2018 and the USA in 2018 by House of Anansi Press Inc.
www.houseofanansi.com

House of Anansi Press is committed to protecting our natural environment.
As part of our efforts, the interior of this book is printed on paper that contains 100% post-
consumer recycled fibres, is acid-free, and is processed chlorine-free.

22 21 20 19 18   1 2 3 4 5

Library and Archives Canada Cataloguing in Publication

Great expectations : twenty-five true stories about childbirth / Lisa
Moore, Dede Crane, editors. — New edition.

Previous edition published under title: Great expectations: twenty-four
true stories about childbirth.
Issued in print and electronic formats.
ISBN 978-1-4870-0389-0 (softcover).—ISBN 978-1-4870-0390-6 (EPUB).—
ISBN 978-1-4870-0391-3 (Kindle)

1. Childbirth. 2. Childbirth—Anecdotes. 3. Childbirth—Popular works.
4. Parent and infant. 5. Authors—Biography. I. Moore, Lisa Lynne, 1964–, editor
II. Crane, Dede, editor

PS8237.C48G74 2018   C814'.6   C2017-904987-C2017-904988-7

Library of Congress Control Number: 2017948421

Series design: Brian Morgan
Cover illustration: Chloe Cushman
Typesetting: Alysia Shewchuk

Canada Council   Conseil des Arts   ONTARIO ARTS COUNCIL
for the Arts   du Canada   CONSEIL DES ARTS DE L'ONTARIO
                                            an Ontario government agency
                                            un organisme du gouvernement de l'Ontario

We acknowledge for their financial support of our publishing program the Canada Council for the Arts,
the Ontario Arts Council, and the Government of Canada through the Canada Book Fund.

Printed and bound in Canada

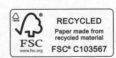

RECYCLED
Paper made from
recycled material
FSC
www.fsc.org   FSC® C103567

To parents past, present, and future

CONTENTS

INTRODUCTION

Emily Urquhart

ON A RAINY DAY last fall, I tucked myself into a carrel at my local library with a copy of *Great Expectations: Twenty-Four True Stories about Childbirth*. The library is where I escape to read and write because even when my two children are absent from our home, their traces — toy-strewn bedrooms, balled-up socks on the couch, art supplies on the kitchen counter — remain tauntingly within reach. I first read this collection after giving birth to my daughter, in that foggy year of early parenthood. I'd fallen, exhausted and grateful, into these childbirth narratives and, wanting to share them, loaned my copy to another new mother. Of course, I never saw it again. So I was looking forward to revisiting these stories on that day in the library, surrounded by stacks of books and fellow readers. After snugging myself into place and diving into the first few essays, however, I was met with a problem I hadn't (but should have) anticipated: I began to weep. It was modest, at first; contained and fairly silent. Then, a line in Esta Spalding's beautiful, sorrowful "Notes from St. Pantaléon" fractured my composure and a sob escaped into the high-ceilinged hush of the library. My carrel-mate, a sixtyish man, who was bespectacled and serious, shifted uncomfortably in his seat. "I'm sorry," I said, shaking my head in a gesture that I hoped assured him that the outburst wouldn't happen again. But of course it did, and soon afterwards I laughed—or rather, I emitted a kind of undignified guffaw. This I blame on Caroline Adderson and her description of the garbage bag of unflattering maternity wear that cycles through generations of pregnant women. (Oh, how I remembered that careworn bag!) The man across from me raised a questioning eyebrow in my direction. I began to wonder if I should sign out one of the library's sound-proof study rooms to continue reading these childbirth stories, just to spare my fellow patrons. I don't know what the serious man was reading, but it certainly wasn't as engaging as the material in my hands.

Few tales can match the drama inherent to childbirth stories, or, as witnessed by my public guffaw, the fierce humour. Yet there are no silly rom-com tropes in these stories. None feature a pregnant woman whose water breaks, Niagara Falls–like, in a high-end dress shop, and there's no comedic hollering at the taxi driver between contractions. Joseph Boyden's memoir of his son's birth does take place in a car, but it's illuminating and harrowing, and the opposite of slapstick. The humour in these essays is deeper, better, relatable, and surprising. Take Edeet Ravel, for example, who writes that her contractions make her feel "that it's the sixteenth century and someone who thinks I'm a witch is trying to extract a confession."

If I could go back, I'd read these stories during rather than after my first pregnancy, when I could have learned my fate from "two tired old warriors going to battle for the last time," as Dede Crane describes herself and her husband, Bill Gaston, when staring down their fourth and final labour experience. Instead, while pregnant, I watched *Orgasmic Birth: The Best Kept Secret*, which depressed me because I knew — deeply, intrinsically — that these women were having babies, not orgasms, and that this video, loaned to me by our bizarre and vaguely qualified doula, was the first in a series of confusing messages about the realities of childbirth. Here, in these pages, we have the (sometimes astonishing) truth. "I realized I had a basement," writes Christine Poutney. "And that's where the pain was coming from." Yes, thank you, tell me more about the basement! And who but Lisa Moore could inform us that the sleep from knock-out painkillers was "so black and cloying, smothering, and absolutely void of sensory detail that I imagine I know what it feels like to be dead."

In these stories I saw glimmers of my own experience, related to the desperation, elation, and mythos of bringing life into the world, but I also marvelled at the tales that didn't mirror my own, as in Afua Cooper's essay, which begins when she is a young woman, new to Canada and its culture, lonely in the midst of her first pregnancy. In turn, I was awed and quieted by the stories that ended differently from my own, such as Lynn Coady's haunting and honest memoir of being a pregnant teenager and choosing adoption because it was the best, if not an easy, choice.

I hope that the (now seasoned) mother who absconded with my first copy of *Great Expectations* passed it on to another reader, as parents have been passing on birth stories since time immemorial. The accoutrements and ideas surrounding birth have changed over the years, but the act, primal and raw, links us to our near and ancient past in a way that nothing else can. It knits us together while also partially remaining a mystery. "We write our stories to make sense of that first breathtaking moment when our children separate from our bodies and begin to become their own individual selves on a journey that takes them away from us," writes Sandra Martin in her essay "Road Trips." For this same reason, I think, we pass these stories onward, laterally, and down, across generations. Also, it's a form of solace. By sharing our birth tales, we learn how none are perfect and that some are traumatic, as Leah McLaren, Karen Connelly, and Curtis Gillespie explore in different but equally compelling ways.

There's another, simpler urge that brings us to share a birth tale, and that's because it's a good story. Gripping and tension-filled, these narratives are the same in that each one will have a beginning, a middle, and an end, but how each story begins and ends, and what happens in-between, occurs in innumerable ways. Expectations are rarely met the way they are imagined. You simply can't predict how a birth will go, just as in these pieces of writing, you can't guess how the author will tell the story.

While re-reading *Great Expectations*, between laughing and weeping, I remembered something my midwife told me just before my second child was born. At a turning point in my labour, when it was time to push my son into this world, she brought our faces close together and we locked eyes. "This will be nothing like the first time," she told me. She might as well have been holding the starter flag at the Grand Prix. It was all I needed to hear to finish that race. My midwife had not been present at my daughter's birth, which had been difficult and fraught. That delivery had happened on a different island, a continent away. I'd relayed the story to her and she had read my medical files, so I assumed that was how she knew that this birth would be unlike my first. I've since changed my mind. I think my midwife could say those words with confidence because she knew that no two birth stories are alike. Each one is a singular miracle, just as each one is a universal tale.

PREFACE

BIRTH IS EVERYBODY'S MIRACLE. There have been billions of human births, so many that one would think it would be a repeated story. How is it, then, that each birth is so unique? Complex, dramatic, full of human strength and frailty, fear, and humour, as well as invaluable wisdom, birth is all the stuff of good stories.

The authors in this collection are some of Canada's finest journalists and fiction writers. They have been shockingly generous in giving us a *felt sense* of what birth demands of us physically, emotionally, and spiritually. Because these authors pull no punches, the stories provide an intuitive map into a landscape that is as much about the practical as the wild.

We wanted first-hand accounts that would be honest about pain and joy. We received stories about the betrayals many of us associate with Western medicine and childbirth. We received stories showing the gratitude many of us felt for medical intervention, for the doctors and nurses who, in some cases, saved our lives or the lives of our children. There are women here who demanded epidurals and were denied them. There are women who wanted natural births and were given epidurals. There are stories of women who felt in control, and those who lost control.

Men who felt outside the experience of birth, even though they wanted desperately to help, and men who were deeply afraid. There are also moments of naked bliss. And there is the kind of poignant humour uncertainty provokes.

These stories cover the spectrum: from a peaceful home birth gone mean to a life-threatening Caesarean to Joseph Boyden's shock as he delivers his son in the back of a Buick Skylark. Caroline Adderson meditates on the absurd realities of pregnancy, and Esta Spalding reminds us of the twinship that birth will always share with death. Bill Gaston shows off his baby-catching skills, while Afua Cooper bridges both cultural and spiritual divides. Jaclyn Moriarty reveals the endurance of mothers through war, earthquake, and heartbreak. Anne Fleming shares how one lesbian couple chooses a donor father. Lynn Coady describes the anguish of giving up a child for adoption, and in the telling, we see the strength and bravery such a decision requires. The list, and the variations on the theme, goes on.

Every parent, together and apart, ventures into sacred and unknowable territory to bring forth a child. Once that child arrives, there is little time to look back. We would like to thank these writers for looking back, for remembering so vividly, for being funny and scared and brave. It has been our great privilege to edit these stories.

Dede Crane and Lisa Moore
March 2008

CONGRATULATIONS, IT'S A TOASTER!

Caroline Adderson

QUITE A NUMBER OF my friends had already had babies by the time I did, none of them easily. One started leaking amniotic fluid and was ordered to check in to Vancouver Women's Hospital, where she had to lie around reading old magazines for months before finally giving birth. Another called me after her delivery to ask that I bring a mirror to the hospital when I visited.

"They don't have mirrors at the hospital?"

"I want to see my hemorrhoid," she said.

When I showed up with flowers and a hand mirror, I saw that her left eye was completely filled with blood.

"You have a hemorrhoid in your *eye*?" I exclaimed.

It was a burst blood vessel. (She paid at both ends, poor thing.) I'd even been in the delivery room and seen the miracle first hand. The friend who invited me — one of the kindest people I know — got rather snippy with the doctor at the crucial moment and passed comment on his breath. I was even more shocked when I laid eyes on the placenta, which I had hitherto imagined as a giant egg white or a benign jellyfish, not a yucky liverish lump. We named it Warren.

You may wonder why I wanted a baby at all after these ruffling experiences. The truth is, if I could have put it off another ten years, I would have, but I was thirty-four. If I waited till I was dying to have a baby, I would probably be dead. So I too signed up for nine months of physical mortification culminating in... Never mind, I'll start with the mortification and save the anticlimax for the end.

THE ONE THING THAT went smoothly for us was the conception. To this day my husband takes absurd pride in the fact that he hit the bull's eye in the first round. As he has so little else to be proud of in the whole birthing process, I refrain from mentioning the *five million* sperm he slung. Four weeks later, I went out and bought a home pregnancy test. There were two sticks to pee on, two chances per kit. I peed on one of the sticks and watched it change colour.

"I'm pregnant," I announced.

"No way," my husband said.

"Yes way." I showed him the stick. He still didn't believe me. He wanted me to pee on the other as a control, as additional proof. But the kit had cost me fifteen dollars, and in a matter of weeks there would be no doubting my condition anyway. Ever thrifty, I gave the leftover stick to a friend.

Like many couples reproducing for the first time, we didn't tell anyone I was pregnant until after I had passed the magic three-month mark. This was to spare us the pain of that second announcement should the pregnancy not come to term. At the time, however, this secrecy seemed like another social convention that ought to go the way of white gloves and pillbox hats, because surely what any woman would want after miscarrying is sympathy. Now that I'm well out of the baby-making business, I feel differently again. The very best time of my pregnancy was those few weeks when I knew I was up the pole yet felt exactly the same. I was pregnant with a secret, with expectation. That schoolyard taunt "I know something you don't know!" was mine to recite silently to everyone I met. It was thrilling. I thought, *This is what a poet feels like when she conceives a perfect line—gloaty and tingly and so superior.* Or so I imagined. I've never written a poem.

Then one morning I woke up not tingly or gloaty at all, but decidedly green. From that point on I was continuously nauseous, though most intensely during the first trimester. Food and food odours made me sicker. I could eat bread, bananas, and Tums, and I ate a lot of bread, bananas, and Tums, because an empty stomach also triggered my nausea. Weirdly, certain visual cues did too. For example, I owned a batik skirt—excellent maternity wear with its drawstring waist—but the pattern on the fabric made me queasy and I had to give it away. I'm very sorry to say (and I apologize sincerely to any readers of Korean heritage) that something about Korean writing also nauseated me. Japanese, Chinese, and Vietnamese script produced no reaction, but every time I passed a Korean restaurant the sign would make me retch.

IN SOME WAYS LIFE was better during the second and third trimesters. I wasn't so intensely nauseous that I had to keep going out of my way to avoid the Korean Presbyterian Church down the street. My stomach, while still iffy, tolerated the occasional non-banana. Then one day, as I stood chatting with a group of teaching colleagues at work, I felt an alarming gush. I hurried to the bathroom and confirmed what I felt: dampness.

At home I told my husband what had happened. "Remember Cheryl?"

"Who?"

"Cheryl. She started leaking. Strict supine bedrest with three-year-old *People* magazines!"

"Oh my God!" my husband said.

We decided that if it happened again, I should call the midwife. It did happen again, a few days later. When I called her, the midwife said it sounded odd but not like leaking amniotic fluid, which would trickle out rather than come in irregular gushes.

"But keep me posted," she said.

The third time it happened, I was at home. I shrieked and my husband came running.

"Smell it," I said.

"Smell what?" he said. "What?"

I was pregnant, so he couldn't refuse. Early on I had suggested he give up alcohol for the duration of the pregnancy, in solidarity with me, but he'd said, "No way." Now he had to do everything I asked. He got down on his knees, balking and cringing before plunging face-first into the crotch of my panties.

"What does it smell like?" I asked. He looked up at me.

"Is it amniotic fluid?"

His look said he was sorry to be the one to tell me. "Sweetheart? It smells like pee."

SOME PEOPLE CLAIM TO find a pregnant woman's body radiantly beautiful and sexy. But if I stuffed a basketball down my shirt, no one would want to have sex with me. My clothes no longer fitted, and I had to dip into the green garbage bag of pastel hand-me-downs passed on by friends and friends of friends. This garbage bag of unflattering, out-of-style maternity wear is as much a fact of pregnancy as edema and Braxton Hicks contractions, and receiving it, a rite of passage. The garments, which never wear out, are eventually returned to the bag to be passed on to the next woman who can't justify the expense of buying clothes she'll wear for only a few months. So these garments circulate in perpetuity. Some cultures believe they are brought to each woman by an evil stork.

While I'm on the subject, let me say a few words about the Maternity Panel. The Maternity Panel — not a meeting of officials from the Ministry of Child and Family Services convened to determine your fitness as a mother — is a polyester semicircle of fabric sewn into maternity clothes where the normal front of the skirt or pants would be. A button is fixed on either side of the panel and wide elastic is threaded through the waistband — usually wizened and unelastic by the time it reaches you. With this system, the waist can be let out buttonhole by buttonhole as you expand, and the polyester can chafe unpleasantly against your tautening belly, and you live in constant fear of your pants falling down in public. The green garbage bag teems with them.

I looked ridiculous by the end of my pregnancy, dressed like a scarecrow, scratching my basketball, crunching my Tums. My face swelled up, giving me grotesquely unsexy beestung lips. Carpal tunnel syndrome numbed me from elbows to fingertips and necessitated that I wear orthotic wrist braces at night. I had a TENS machine too, for the back pain, as well as an extra pillow under my knees. I already wore a mouthguard because I grind my teeth, and earplugs because my husband snores. Then I got bronchitis, which made the gushing problem a lot worse. I wondered if it was really worth it. Really.

"Are you worth it? Yeah, you. Hello? Hello?"

I knocked. Amazingly, he answered. If I knocked, he knocked back. We could, I discovered, communicate perfectly. "One kick for yes, two for no. Are you worth it? Yes or no?"

One swift kick. "Naturally *you'd* think so."

Communicating with my unborn son was the best thing about being pregnant: I had an oracle living inside me. Throughout my last trimester he predicted the weather, counselled me on my life and career, and helped make all the day-to-day decisions. I sought his opinion on everything. Some days I would picture him as a smiling weatherman, others as Ann Landers or a bearded dwarf in a toga and sandals—each of these in miniature, curled fetal and suspended upside down.

WE NEVER MANAGED TO make a birth plan. I did read the manuals, though my husband wouldn't. (He's anti-DIY. He won't even mow the lawn.) But he couldn't get out of taking the childbirth course. No way. He attended and was the only person in the class who shouted during the video. As the baby came cannonballing out, he lunged forward with a "Whoa, Nelly!" Everyone tittered and shifted slightly away from us.

Three and a half weeks before my due date, the midwives scheduled our first home visit. During it we were going to discuss our birth plan, including, I hoped, how to keep my husband from embarrassing me. The day before, I realized I didn't have anything to offer the midwives with their tea.

"Should I get some cookies?"

One kick.

"Okay. Let's go."

I trundled the five blocks to the store and the five blocks back. I could barely walk by that point.

That evening I told my husband, a night owl, that he should

start catching up on his sleep. I said he should come to bed early. He didn't. (Who can blame him, with the Bride of Frankenstein taking up most of the bed?) He tucked himself in around two. A few hours later I woke thinking, "Lordy, I've *really* wet myself now." I'd wet the whole bed with amniotic fluid, and we didn't have a birth plan.

After a few phone calls, a Caesarean was hastily arranged, which was neither unexpected nor disappointing. I remembered what my friends had gone through — the bloody eye, the snippy mouth — and decided I'd already suffered enough. The other reason I was grateful for the Caesarean was that I happened to be in the planning stage of a novel in which one of the main characters is paralyzed from the waist down. I was going to have a baby *and* do research at the same time! Still, I was nervous and demanded to know the stats: how many people have been left permanently paralyzed by a spinal block? Hardly any, I was reassured. I consulted my personal oracle and learned he was rather anxious to get out.

By the time we got to the hospital, the contractions were a couple of minutes apart and very, very painful, yet when the doctor examined me he said I wasn't even dilated.

"What? Not at all?"

When the anesthetist showed up, I tried to kiss his hand.

I remember the needle going into my back, and another gush — spinal fluid this time. Then there was heaviness, but no pain. Someone erected a fabric screen across my waist so I wouldn't be able to see what was going on. My bleary husband was banished to the other side with me, where he couldn't make trouble. The doctor's and intern's caps and masks poked up over the top of the screen like a puppet show. The doctor was telling the intern what to do. *Great*, I thought, *a beginner*. And since cutting and stitching were involved, I couldn't help but think of my first, failed sewing project in Grade 7 with the two left sleeves. I rolled my eyes and saw the light above us, which had a wide chrome rim. I could watch everything they were doing in the rim of the light. There I was, *wide open*. I shut my eyes.

The upper part of my body, the part that had feeling, was being jostled back and forth. It was as if the numb part of me was a sack someone was reaching into to remove whatever was inside. It seemed to be stuck, and now I pictured the object inside me as having corners, making it difficult to remove from a full sack. A toaster. The doctor was murmuring encouragement to the intern, warning him about the cord. The cord of the toaster. *How absurd*, I thought. *All along I've been talking to a toaster.* Then they exclaimed on the other side of the screen, and on our side my husband said, "Oh. It's a boy," quietly, in the sweetest tone, so I knew that all along this was what he had been hoping for. Someone raised him above the screen so I could see him—my son, runty, nearsighted, incontinent mess that he was. Not a toaster at all. You just don't instantly love a kitchen appliance.

THE NEXT DAY THE midwife came to see me. I shook my fist at her. "You lied!"

"Lied?"

"You never told me how much it would hurt."

"Why would I?" she said. "Nothing I could say would prepare you for it."

Before I had a baby, I used to think there was a reason women suffered to have a child. I thought the pain and discomfort were some kind of test. If you got through that, then the rest of it— the diapers, the sleeplessness, the boredom, the unreciprocated baby talk—would seem easy. I also believed that the physical pain was somehow connected to a mother's ability to love. No pain, no love. This is twaddle, of course. Just ask any adoptive parent. What no midwife or obstetrician can really prepare you for is the intensity of that love.

My son is eight now. Sometimes I'll play the old game. "Pancakes for breakfast? Yes or no? Yes or no?"

"Mom," he'll say, "stop poking me."

He doesn't remember. Or does he? The mere sight of a banana makes him gag.

Even now we can hardly believe this wonderful person came from us. We *made* him. Us? How?

Because all the truisms — that you'll forget the pain, that you'll love your child more than yourself — turned out to be true. I'd do anything for my child. Anything. Even give birth to him.

NOTES FROM ST. PANTALÉON

Esta Spalding

INDUSTRIOUS AS A FORENSIC team, the bees in the lavender bush outside the limestone house search for pollen. Nothing will deter them. Not the wind, which is so strong that it carries the voices of the labourers in the vineyard half a mile down the hill. Driving up the dirt road yesterday, I stopped for a moment to watch this mysterious work. What are the labourers doing now, when hints of green are just beginning to emerge from the gnarled, half-dead stumps of the winter vines? Are they pruning so soon, already cutting those tender shoots?

A gust of wind parts the grass, suddenly revealing the child's rubber ball, missing since early this afternoon. I'd searched for it, but to no avail. There were tears and then, suddenly, there was sleep. She slept on my shoulder.

What happiness to carry her upstairs, to feel the weight that sleep seemed to add to her little body, to lay her down in the crib. Now, seeing the blue ball there in the grass, I want to wake her, watch her face burst into delight as I place it in her tiny raccoon hands. Say to her, See, you don't have to worry, what is lost, returns.

SHE WAS BORN TWO years before in a hospital in Vancouver. Gemma, we named her. Because we liked the sound of it, suggesting a gem or jewel. And because it seemed to fit—to sound right—with her difficult, odd last name. Only later, when we looked it up, did we see that the name's root meant "bud" and was the origin of *Gemini*, the twins. By then it was too late to change.

In the first photograph of her—an ultrasound—her arm seems to be around the waist of her twin. Hugging, the nurse said.

AT FIFTEEN WEEKS I BEGIN to bleed. This is not unusual for me. I have had two miscarriages in the past two years, and so from my experience this is what pregnancy is. You miss your period. You get excited. You begin to make all the plans. What time of year will the child be born? Will I quit work, take a leave? What will my new life be? You get sick. The nausea is comforting—it means the pregnancy is going well, the baby developing properly, doesn't it? Only it doesn't mean that at all. When you begin to bleed and the feeling of labour comes at twelve or thirteen weeks, you learn that it will be only a matter of time before the pregnancy that was never a baby (you keep reminding yourself of this) is gone.

And this time is the same.

The bleeding begins. That you are pregnant with twins, that they each have a heartbeat—something that never developed in either of the other two pregnancies—seems to you not to matter. You assume you are going to miscarry again. There is no way to prepare for this. It is devastating. A massive grief multiplied by two.

You try not to dwell on it. You rent *The Forsyte Saga*—three generations, two wars, six hours of drama; you assume that by the time it's over the pregnancy will be too. But lo and behold, it isn't. Instead there's an ultrasound. One of the babies—Twin A, the doctors call her—is developing properly. The other—Twin B—has an *abrupted placenta*. This means the placenta isn't properly attached to the wall of the uterus; nutrients aren't getting to the fetus; the fetus's growth has been stunted. And worse: the doctors fear that the bleeding from Twin B's placenta will irritate the uterus and cause early labour. Not only will Twin B be lost, but Twin A will be born too early, before she has a chance of surviving. The doctors tell you to lie down and not get up until the bleeding stops. And so you get in bed and you stay in bed for what turns out to be sixteen weeks.

———

LIKE SO MUCH ELSE in our lives since Gemma's birth, for D. and me this trip to France is different than any vacation we took during the ten years we were together without a child. Instead of visiting art galleries and historical museums, we push Gemma in her stroller through the park, ride merry-go-rounds, and eat frites, taking hundreds of pictures of her ketchup-spattered face. Instead of staying in hotels, we rent a house and we spend a lot of time out in the yard naming the animals we meet. By day there are crickets, butterflies, praying mantises, and bunnies; by evening, snails, owls, and bats. We plot our excursions to various medieval hilltop towns not by the beauty of their stone carvings or stained-glass cathedrals, but by the quality of their ice cream shops and crepe stands. In Avignon we walk on the bridge, the famous *pont*. It delights Gemma to discover that the bridge goes only halfway across the river. We ask and are told that the other half was routinely destroyed by floods until it was finally abandoned. After that, one supposes, the bridge fell out of use for everything but dancing.

"L'on y danse, l'on y danse," we sing to Gemma, dancing on the bridge, holding on to our hats — and the child — for fear they may blow away.

I LIE IN BED FOR those sixteen weeks. Mostly reading or doing email. Talking on the phone. Mostly resisting watching daytime TV. I sleep a lot.

A recurring daydream from that time: I am floating on a raft in a magnificent river, on either side of which are high limestone walls. The walls are pockmarked with small clefts and in the clefts are the delicate nests of cliff swallows. Sometimes in the dream I watch the swallows flit across the river, chasing insects, carrying their prey back to the nests, to the hungry throats waiting there. Other times, from my bed on the raft I see no birds and am aware that the nests on the cliffs are empty, that they've been abandoned years before. That they are merely a delicate, desiccated lace decorating the cliff face.

For days at a time I lie on the raft — sometimes awake and sometimes asleep — but always dreaming that the tips of my fingers are dragging in the river. Always aware of the twins, their thoughtless undulations, inside me. Always utterly still for fear one twin will come unmoored and slip from its berth, crossing the river without me.

And while I sleep and dream, D. does everything else. He shops, cooks, cleans, takes out the trash. He goes to work and brings home news of the world beyond the bedroom walls. He makes me the egg sandwiches that I crave: two fried eggs tucked between two slices of bread.

I lie there on my back, eating the sandwiches and making promises to myself. I will do this thing perfectly — lie still perfectly — for five months or six months, if only someday I will be able to hold them. Or at least hold one of them.

⁓

ONE NIGHT THE BLEEDING begins again in earnest. We go to the hospital. Now that we are at twenty-six weeks the doctors treat me differently. Though Twin B is still considered too small to survive, Twin A is viable. And so I am admitted to the hospital. There's nothing they can do to help the babies or to stop the bleeding, but if I'm in the hospital I'm close to the doctors and the equipment necessary to save Twin A.

D. goes home. I go to sleep in my white room, listening to the breathing of the woman in the bed beside me — another obstetrical oddity — who periodically wakes up during the night to go out onto the roof and smoke. I can't help wondering if this is part of the reason for the problems with her pregnancy. But this is the kind of blame-the-mother thinking that I try to avoid. It's the kind of thinking that wakes me in the middle of the night, desperate with guilt: I am a woman who isn't feeding her child. All those egg sandwiches and still my body is failing Twin B. The baby isn't getting what it needs from me.

One night I wake in the darkness to see a nurse bent over me, checking the fetal heart-rate monitors that are attached to my enormous belly. She apologizes for waking me, tells me that both babies still have heartbeats, and then she sits down on the edge of the bed to tell me about her daughter. Jenna is her name and she is retarded. The nurse uses this word: *retarded*. She tells me about Jenna's life and about how challenging it is both for Jenna and for her. She tells me it is rewarding too. Hard, but rewarding. She wouldn't want any other daughter. She says this twice, then she says she finds strength from other parents who have similar children. If Twin B survives, she tells me, she and those other parents will be there for me.

It is only after she's left that I understand what she is telling me. Eliot, we call this child (we don't yet know if it is a boy or a girl, because it's so tiny that even on the detailed ultrasound the doctors can't discern the sex).

But I don't see this nurse again, and a few days later the bleeding stops and I go back to my bed at home.

THE ENGINE IDLES. MY foot's on the brake. There's a horse a few yards away, chewing dandelions and staring at us through an electric fence. Gemma, in her car seat, has asked me for juice and I've pulled over onto the gravel shoulder of a road through the town called St. Pantaléon. Now she wants to get out and touch the horse, to name him as has become our ritual with all the animals we meet, but I'm too afraid of her touching the fence and so I tell her we have to just look from the car. While she studies the horse and he studies her, I unzip the backpack on the passenger seat and pull out a bottle of apricot juice. I pour some into her sippy cup and then turn to her in the back — feeling the engine roar as I accidentally hit the gas pedal. Luckily the automatic transmission is in Park and so we don't lurch forward, but the sudden roar is enough to get me to turn the engine off while she drinks her juice. Besides, we're not in a rush. We've been to Gordes to eat ice cream and chase pigeons through the narrow cobblestone streets. She's had a nap in the car and we are on our way back to the limestone house, where D. has asked for the afternoon alone to work on a research paper. And it is a lovely little village, St. Pantaléon. The closest place to the limestone house we're staying in. It's so small there's no café or grocery, just a church and few old stone houses built close enough together to give the place a name on the map. I decide we should have a walk—electric fence or not—and so we get out of the car and toddle hand in hand to the only place there is to go: the church.

I remember it like this: blue light through the stained glass. A church comforting in its emptiness. The single white candle (burning in front of a painting of Mary and the infant Jesus) signals that the place is inhabited, that it's necessary to someone. This is comforting too.

I give Gemma a coin and she puts it in the slot and together we light another candle, leaving it for someone else to find. It's as we're leaving that I see the small pamphlet describing the history of St. Pantaléon, of this church built to accommodate the graves of children who died before they could be baptized, the graves of children who were *in limbo*. The priest of St. Pantaléon was given the task of naming and baptizing these souls so they too could ascend to heaven.

———

AT THIRTY-ONE WEEKS TWIN A is doing very well. She—we now know she is a she—is growing normally, and from the ultrasounds the doctors estimate that she is probably over three pounds. Twin B, though still alive (and still not revealing his or her sex), is not growing as the doctors would like. There appear to be some oddities in the development of the brain, and the baby's weight is closer to a pound, the normal weight of a fetus at twenty-four weeks. I now have nurses stopping by the house every few days to check on the babies' heart rates and to monitor the strange "false labour" contractions that began a week ago. These visits are painful to me, not just because I'm the focus of so much unwanted attention but also because, as with everything else about this pregnancy, I completely lack control. I can't even offer the nurses a cup of tea or coffee, as I'm not allowed out of bed to make it. The nurse is concerned that I'm going into labour, and I'm scheduled for an ultrasound that day. Because my mother is flying into Vancouver and because the hospital is near the airport, I'm allowed to break my routine to pick up my mother from her flight. And so I find myself standing—on my own two feet!—at the baggage claim, watching the enormous machine giving birth to its planeload of luggage.

I hear a familiar voice calling my name and turn to see a colleague—a friend, really—whom I haven't seen in more than a year. He's someone I've worked with as a writer on a couple of different TV shows. We hug. He admires my belly, and I'm suddenly aware of how few people have seen it, of how not used to being in public I am, of how narrow the boundaries of my life have become. A moment later my mother is there, pulling me into her arms, touching my stomach. Amazed by it too. I am an apartment building, or at least a room for lease.

My mother goes with me to the hospital, where I'm given an ultrasound. Everything is the same: Twin A looking good and growing, Twin B not so much—still under a pound. The nurse is sympathetic, but this kind of news is routine for her. She doesn't know me. And so she turns on the lights and tells me I can put on my clothes and go home. I'll have another ultrasound scheduled for two weeks from now. "You're doing a good job," she says, "You've gotten them this far," though both of us know I have very little to do with the outcome. But it's this little hint of empathy on her part that allows me to ask, "What about the false labour?" She doesn't know what I'm talking about. "I've been having these contractions. The nurses wanted me to get checked out. If you could just check my cervix." I don't know where this instinct to be pushy comes from, but so often in my life it's gotten me into terrible trouble (as my friend from the TV shows would agree). In this case it saves me. It saves us. Because the nurse's inspection reveals that my cervix is dilated; I am hours away from full-blown labour. If I'd gone home, the babies would've been born there. No doctors, no equipment, no chance. Instead I'm ushered into the labour suite, hooked up to monitors. Sometime later, a stout doctor with bright eyes and a ready grin appears and tells us — D. and my mother are with me now — that he suspects the birth will happen that night. (Doesn't time move strangely in the hospital? Hours go by in a rush, and then one intense minute seems to last all night.) He tells us we have a decision to make: we need to decide whether or not to monitor Twin B's heartbeat.

You see, he says, babies under a pound never survive so it's very possible Twin B will suffer during the labour and expire (does he really say *expire* or do I just imagine this?). But this isn't his main concern. He implies that Twin B's not surviving labour would be the result of Twin B's not having developed properly; he stresses that this is how nature works. His main concern is that if we monitor Twin B we will make decisions based on Twin B's heart rate and not on the health of Twin A. He wants us to focus on Twin A. On Gemma. On what will be best for her. And to leave Twin B to fate. No, not to fate — those are my words.

"Let nature take its course," is what he says with those impossibly twinkly eyes and that Chesire cat grin. We have to decide.

And so we think. To monitor Twin B or not? The hours seem to pass without our counting them. And suddenly it's almost midnight and the labour is intense. I remember being on all fours. I remember being stretched over a yoga ball. I remember we hadn't yet decided anything. I remember the pain. I remember ice in my mouth and a rock-solid nurse talking me through each wave as it came.

And in the middle of this I remember a pediatrician telling us he thought the other doctors were wrong. Maybe there wouldn't be brain damage, maybe the ultrasounds were all incorrect. Maybe Twin B had a chance of surviving because, though the fetus was less than a pound (less than four sticks of butter), it was thirty-one weeks, and those weeks of growth might have made our second baby stronger than other babies of that size. We'd talked to other pediatricians during the pregnancy, but never one who said anything like this. I remember my doctor of the bright eyes and the grin suddenly not smiling, suddenly furious at this other doctor's intrusion. I remember him pointedly stating that if Twin B did survive, we — not the pediatrician — were the ones who would have to raise this "damaged" child. And I suddenly loved him for saying this, for giving us a pass if we wanted it, for making it okay to "focus only on Twin A." But it was too late. D.'s eyes had lit up at the pediatrician's words — he wanted so badly to believe — and I knew the light in D.'s eyes meant we would have to do everything to save Twin B. That if we didn't our marriage would always have that in it. That seed of resentment. There would always be between us the understanding that we could have done more to save our littlest baby.

The pediatrician's suggestion was reckless. Making decisions about the delivery based on a baby who had almost no chance of surviving might put Twin A at risk. Much, much later we saw this pediatrician posturing in front of news cameras, the lead doctor for a set of sextuplets born at the same hospital. And we wondered then, was his treatment of us all about headlines? Was he trying to be the delivery jockey who kept alive the "only baby under a pound ever to survive"? But we didn't consider this at the time. Instead we took his reckless suggestion. We put the heart monitor on Twin B. We decided to do everything we could to make sure Twin B survived the labour. And just a moment or two after we began to monitor it, the baby's heart rate plummeted. It had begun to suffer from the contractions. If the labour continued, Twin B was going to lose all oxygen. To *expire*.

"If you want to save the baby, you have to have an emergency C-section." The grin was gone, the face utterly serious. "Things will happen very fast." I looked at D. and he nodded yes.

MINUTES LATER I AM ON the table, being cut open. They've put a needle in my spine and rubbed ice on my belly, and the second I can't feel it, my doctor with the knife says, "Cut," and he slices in. I see myself almost from above. Like a plane crash. The scorched earth of a field, the sheared-off wings, the fuselage. He is tunnelling in, this brave doctor. He is going to pull out the survivors.

"HERE'S YOUR BABY GIRL." He lifts a bloody, wet, squalling creature from my belly and holds her up for me to see before handing her to the pediatrician. I know without being told that Gemma is fine, and I feel a rush of the purest pleasure flush through me. All those weeks of waiting. All those promises. And she is here. Pulled from thin air. Wet, noisy, alive.

I see him lift a second bundle from out of my belly and hand it off to the pediatrician — to the team that is assembled around the incubator. "Is he okay?" I'm shouting. I realize I've always assumed Twin B is a boy. "They're working on her," D says. Her?

I could not have seen them pushing on her little lungs, trying to coax the oxygen into them, trying to get her to breathe. But I feel that I saw it. Did D. narrate it to me? Impossible to imagine that he would be able to do that. So how do I know what happened? How do I have these images? How do I know that they worked on her lungs, that she would not breathe, that she would not take that gulp of air required to live?

D. WENT WITH GEMMA (in her little incubator on wheels) to the intensive care nursery. I was stitched up and wheeled on my bed into the recovery room. The doctor, the lovely Chesire-cat doctor, put Eliot, swaddled, into my arms. A little girl. My little girl. Dead now. How I held on to her like a child clutching a favourite doll. (Though she was not like a doll at all. She was so unbeautiful. Her shrivelled head and wrinkled skin. Her blueness. And swaddled as though there were any way to protect her against that cold.) How I loved her, and knew that if she'd lived I would've loved her no matter what.

LATER, STILL ON MY bed, still holding Eliot, I am wheeled into the intensive care nursery to see Gemma. I peer at her in her brightly lit nest. She is as small as a baby chick you'd hold in your palm at Eastertime. They open the oval door of her incubator and I put my hand inside. Though she'd been asleep, she wakes, opens her eyes, and with her little hand she grips my finger. She holds on to me. That little raccoon hand holds on to me.

Never in my life more joy.
And the dead child in my arms: such sorrow.
Joy and sorrow. Twins.

———

THE SKY IS DARKENING. The bats come out, flitting through the air above the pear tree and out in the direction of the vineyard, riding the thin breeze over the vines. Inside the limestone house a light goes on and I hear D. talking to Gemma about dinner. I am still outside, reading the little pamphlet from the church in St. Pantaléon, wondering if we see a pattern in something because we want to see a pattern or because there is a pattern to see.

Suddenly there are headlights in the driveway. A man pulling up, getting out of his car. He steps towards me, asking, "Vous êtes perdue?" I think for a moment. Is this one of those French phrases that mean something else? He must be telling me that he is lost. But no. He repeats it again, "Vous êtes perdue?" Are you lost?

I hesitate.

From inside I hear Gemma calling me. "Mama," she says, "come inside."

"Non." I tell him. "Pas du tout."

He disappears like the ghost he might be.

I look above me where Gemini is just now appearing in the night sky. Someday she will ask me, what if it had gone differently? I won't have the answer then either. I can tell her we need the darkness to see the stars. I can say that much. And I can go inside to her. My daughter. I can go inside.

LANDINGS

Dede Crane

THE BABY MOVES INSIDE my pregnant belly and a small but solid-looking lump pushes out just under a rib. A heel? I place two fingers against the tiny bulge and it instantly responds with a push. I push, it pushes back. I push, it pushes back. Because of this back-and-forth communication, I know this one's a girl. In my experience, boys don't possess this understanding of otherness, of separation.

My children, eleven, nine, and five, are asleep. My husband, Bill, is too. My youngest child started school nine months ago. My oldest is a year away from her first menstruation. I am forty, my husband forty-six. This child I'm carrying will be our "bonus baby," as somebody kind once put it.

Due any day now, I too should be in bed. But I'm energized and stay up sorting the storage room, deciding what stays and what goes. We sold the house today. Signed the final papers. We are leaving in a month to fly across this wide-hipped country to British Columbia and a dental plan. There is another mouth on its way. We can really use a dental plan.

I'm excited about the move, feel ready for a change, but have trouble with the getting there. I'm deeply, viscerally afraid of flying. How something that leaden can fly makes no practical sense to me. And this time all my precious cargo will be together in that one improbable machine...I think of my friend Cathy, who mocks my fear. She loves planes.

"Look at the odds," she says.

I do. Trust me. If there's been a recent plane crash in the news—the bigger, the better—I am morbidly relieved, believing my odds are drastically improved.

The benign Braxton Hicks contractions make a jerk-like leap to something with ambition, intent, and it shocks my nervous system awake. Here we go again. It's just after midnight. I should have slept. I make my way upstairs.

———

A YEAR AND A day ago, when her labour began, Cathy had stopped by. It was early afternoon. Since it was her second go around, she was more excited than nervous. Her pregnancy had gone smoothly; she was bigger than last time: an excess of amniotic fluid, she was told, but nothing to be concerned about. She didn't stay long, said she'd call me and keep me posted, that she was looking forward to losing some weight today. I laughed. Cathy could always make me laugh.

"Keep moving," was my advice to her.

She had a son, Nicholas, five years old and best friends with my five-year-old. We'd both daydreamed she'd have a girl this time. Had named her Mollie. Black hair, round eyes like her mother. A talker.

THE ROADS ARE EMPTY on our short drive to Everett Chalmers Hospital. Spring is marking out territory, and the air through the open window is fragrant and moist. I breathe through another contraction, press a hand against the dash and distract myself with familiar passing landscapes. Bill keeps his eyes ahead. He understands not to look at me during a contraction, not to speak unless spoken to. I know he is utterly attuned to my every movement, listening for clues about my well-being, my wish his command. I am so grateful not to have to explain myself.

The discomfort of the contractions is familiar. My belly slowly seizes, grows rock-hard, becomes a boulder-sized charley horse the rest of my body tenses against. The contraction peaks, then gradually releases me. Releases us. I wonder how this fist-like squeeze is experienced by the baby. It can't feel good.

By child number four I understand labour's stages, its varying strengths. These contractions are doable.

My last labour was only four and a half hours. Because it was back labour, I gave birth on hands and knees, rump in the air. The baby emerged face up, his large eyes squinting at the sudden brightness and my husband's looming face.

"Hello, there. Who are you?" My husband's voice was awed, teary, as he cradled the blinking head in his gloved hand. We still didn't know the baby's sex. "The baby's alert... listening," he told me, the freak with heads at opposite ends.

This child still likes to make an amusing entrance, and we still ask ourselves, *Who are you?*

Labour with my second child, at Grace Maternity, took eleven hours. When the head emerged, the doctor announced in a strange sing-song, "The cord's around the neck." It was a teacherly voice and I could feel the interns staring, bug-eyed. The doctor paused for three time-lapsed seconds. "And it comes off easily," she continued and the room breathed again.

I picture the white calm of our son's face as two nurses rubbed him alive. I recall a single, forced squawk. Even now this boy is too laid-back for tears, for making a fuss.

My first labour, though, was an endurance test and a near plane crash. On my initial visit to the OB office here in Fredericton, pregnant with my third—another new city, another new doctor—a stern, harried nurse ordered me onto the scales, checked my blood pressure, and then got down to obtaining pertinent background information.

"How long was your first labour?"

"Fifty hours," I said, proud that I'd gotten her to stop mid-agenda and look up from her clipboard. Her lips parted with what I imagined was sympathy, even admiration. I was ready to tell my story, how my blood pressure had soared, the baby two weeks early and not quite ready . . .

"No, it wasn't," she said, as if scolding a child for its perverse imagination.

It was my turn to stop. "Well, from my first labour pain I couldn't sleep and they came every—"

"I'm not putting down fifty," she interrupted.

"Put whatever you like," I said. My breathing had become shallow.

I stole a look at my chart later. She had written down twenty, not even half of fifty.

My first birth: I'd hoped to have a home birth, but after forty hours of hard, sleepless labour, my midwife suggested we head to the hospital, Toronto East General. Even after my water was forcibly broken, I was still only three centimetres dilated. Without the Pitocin drip, without an epidural, I don't believe I would have survived. Her body was born tense, her head cranked to one side. She had a fist pressed to her mouth as she uttered a tense cry. From all that compression her head was shaped like a fat banana. The doctor assured us this shape was temporary. We'd laugh about it later. Tease her about it, our intense daughter, the high achiever, always ahead of schedule.

Here in the car, I realize I'm relieved that only Bill is accompanying me to the hospital. For all my other births we had a midwife along, a person paid to be in charge. For the third birth, the two-headed one, we also brought along my mother. My mother was dressed in white linen slacks and a striped navy and white top with matching handbag. She had never witnessed a birth, not even of her own children. General anesthesia was standard procedure in the fifties, and my mother is still thankful to have been unconscious for all three of her children's arrivals. Later that day, after my son was born, my mother had compared the sight of her panting daughter with a small head poking out of her backside to the rocket launch she'd witnessed at Cape Canaveral.

"Now *that* was something," she said, meaning the rocket launch.

We park in the pay lot and together walk up to the front doors of the hospital. The quiet is surreal. The usual traffic at the entryway — folks in wheelchairs, visitors coming and going, patients and employees stepping outside to smoke — doesn't exist. There is nobody at reception to greet us. The lights are dimmed. No security guard. We look at each other. The last people on earth. We continue towards the elevator but I have to stop and press the wall. My groan fills the silence, washes down the empty hallways. Nobody comes. This child was wholly unexpected, and nine months earlier we had wavered, had wondered what we should do. We'd considered options.

"Okay," I say as the contraction subsides, and we continue. The elevator is also empty. Bill watches the floor's numbers light up as we ascend. He yawns but has the decency to cover his mouth. Our eyes meet. Here we are again. Two tired old warriors going to battle for the last time.

A YEAR AND A day ago, it was dark out when Cathy called and told me we were wrong. It was a boy, fair-haired, with his father's long face and her eyes.

"He's gorgeous," she said. "We named him Anton."

Her relief was palpable. She said her water broke like a dam, the nurse slipping and nearly breaking her neck.

"Anton," I repeated.

"He was having trouble breastfeeding," she said. "Couldn't breathe through his nose properly, so they've taken him to clear out his passages, check his lungs. They think he swallowed some of my ocean." She laughed her brisk laugh, then asked me to call our mutual friends and let them know.

WE ARRIVE AT A dimly lit maternity ward. But there is a body at reception, who greets us in a hushed voice. I imagine sleeping babies around the corner or a row of exhausted doctors, all curled up, thumbs curiously close to their slung-open mouths, doctors desperate for uninterrupted...

We're escorted to our room by a petite middle-aged nurse

who gives me meek glances, assessing her evening's work.

"This is my fourth child," I say, letting her off the hook. She nods knowingly. "I'm here if you need anything."

I have to pause in the narrow hall, press the wall, and concentrate now on being bigger than the pain, which has turned spiteful. We pass the maternity lounge, where a young couple is holding hands, watching TV. Canned laughter erupts from the screen but the couple don't break a smile. A yoga ball, turquoise green, sits in the corner of the room. I want it. I ask the nurse if I can have it.

Yes.

Bill carries the ball. It's the least he can do.

I set myself up on the ball, which feels roomy and forgiving under my pelvis. I rock my bones. I rock my baby. Imagine things opening down there and making way. I lay my exhausted upper body on the tall, narrow bed. It's three in the morning. I really should have slept. The nurse asks if I want nitrous oxide. Though it has never worked for me before, I say sure. As she leaves to fetch the laughing gas, Bill asks, real nice, if I'd like him to rub my back the way I wanted for labours one and two. No. He jokes about wrestling me for first go at the laughing gas. I can smile but I can't laugh. I am alone in this, so very alone, and need all my focus for what lies ahead.

———

A YEAR AGO, I CALLED Cathy, who had just given birth in this very hospital. I was hoping to go visit and meet Anton. Her tone was matter-of-fact and defensive.

"There's something wrong with the baby," she said.

In an instant he had lost his name.

"A muscular disorder. Genetic," she added, pointing fingers. "His lungs can't function on their own. He doesn't have the ability to nurse and they don't think he'll live."

"Oh, Cathy," I said and burst out crying.

And after thirty seconds passed, so did she.

⌒

MY DOCTOR'S PARTNER, A man I've never laid eyes on, comes in with the nitrous oxide. He tells me that my doctor, the one with whom I've worked hard at developing a meaningful relationship over the past nine months, is in *Bermuda*, of all places. I don't understand why I wasn't informed of his vacation plans. Dr. So-and-so shakes my hand, my husband's hand. He has sleep-wrecked hair. He sits down and takes his time teaching me how to use the gas, explains that it works only if you breathe it in well ahead of a contraction, using deep, even breaths.

"Don't wait until a contraction begins. That's too late." He sounds experienced. He leaves then. Goes back to bed.

Riding my ball, I lay my upper body back down on the bed, turn my head to the side, and hold the gas mask to my face. I draw nothing but nitrous oxide into my lungs in deep yoga breaths. I have read that laughing gas increases oxygen in the blood, that it doesn't slow labour or harm the baby. I hope it's true, because the next contraction doesn't hurt. Could it be? Ball, bed, and laughing gas, contractions come and go. No big deal. It's a miracle. Why had no one ever taught me how to use this stuff before? I want to announce my labour cure to the world, but refuse to remove the mask from my mouth. I listen to the nurse and Bill talk of things I instantly forget. I labour away, painlessly.

Other than to check the heartbeat, the nurse is content to

ignore me. My husband is a nice guy, a girl's-best-friend type, and easy to talk to. They chat on.

Two hours later the next contraction has me pounding the bed.

"Transition time?" asks the nurse, slowly paying attention.

The next contraction is off the charts.

"It's too much," I pant, shaking my head and slapping at the bed, the air, the ball.

My round throne is removed, that worthless gas wheeled away, and Dr. So-and-so is summoned. I'm up on the tall, narrow bed. Lights and action. Bill is saying all the right things and I believe him: "It's almost over. Our baby's coming. It's almost over." He is a professional by now, yet there is apprehension in his voice too. No one can predict the future.

———

A YEAR AGO, I ARRIVED on this same floor to see Cathy. I didn't bring flowers. It didn't seem right. She was in her room pumping her milk because a nurse had told her to. The baby was in the intensive care nursery. There was a hard sadness in her face. I kissed her forehead and tears involuntarily started down my face.

"Don't," she told me. Cathy was too practical for sympathy. She said she would not take me to see the baby because she couldn't bear to see or hold him for fear of bonding with him, of loving him. Her husband, Tilmann, and Nicholas, her five-yearold, would take me. She ordered me not to cry around Nicholas. I promised.

Her sick baby was a puppet hung by tubes and needles, hooked up to machines and beeping monitors. His head was shaved where one of the needles pierced his scalp; a bandage covered his miniature thigh where a plug of flesh had been removed for diagnostic testing. Cathy's elegant and soft-spoken husband, a professor of marine biology, expressed hopeful things to me in front of Nicholas: "He'll have to stay in the hospital for a while so they can run tests and find out what's wrong. Then he can get stronger."

We looked on, helpless, at this child under glass.

"I'm a big brother now," Nicholas informed me.

"You sure are, Nicholas," I said, and quickly excused myself in order to weep in the other room.

———

THE FIRST URGE TO push subsumes my body and my will. The downward pull of gravity has multiplied a hundredfold. I am giving birth to a horse. I lie on my right side, just because. I'm making what my funny husband will later describe as rhino mating calls. I have no choice but to surrender, to trust this alien body, this pain, this doctor I've just met tonight.

The crowning is a branding ring of fire, and I yell at this last child, just like I yelled at each one before, "Get out! Get out!" A mother's first words.

The head is out in just two pushes. The worst now over.

The body follows easily on the next contraction. *Flubbidy-flub*, loose limbs and slippery skin. That's how it always feels to me. *Flubbidy-flub*. The doctor lets Bill catch the baby, knowing he's experienced at this, and will have him cut the cord.

As the baby is wiped off she makes gusty, unapologetic cries. She knows what she likes and doesn't. This one's a decision maker. In my arms she quiets and we look at each other, push back and forth with our gaze. I'm struck by the architecture of her eyebrows. Two stunningly graceful arcs.

"Hello, sweetheart," I say as she roots for my breast.

Bill's face is beside mine, his breath warm on my neck as his arms reach around me and around her. I can include him now, appreciate him all over again. We are smiling tired. The battle over. Not won, not lost, just over.

CATHY IS MY FIRST guest. She has brought me flowers, orange tiger lilies. Yesterday her Anton, who has only recently come home from the hospital, had his first birthday. Cathy has learned to feed him her breast milk through a tube inserted in his stomach. She suctions his tiny lungs every three hours to ward off the ever-present threat of pneumonia, and has developed a hawk's eye for changes in his colour or mood. She has been in contact with other parents whose children have this rare neuromuscular disorder, has learned things she never had any desire to know. Her life is completely changed.

"Can I hold her?" Cathy asks.

Propped up in bed, I hand her my baby girl, proud but guilty.

"She's perfect," she says, her eyes too bright.

I have a ridiculous but vivid image of her dropping my child on the cement floor, and quickly shut it down.

"Four kids, eh?" she says, shaking her head as she hands back my baby. "You poor bugger."

——

FOUR WEEKS AFTER GIVING birth, I fly with my four children, husband, and a dog to Vancouver Island. On the plane I breastfeed obsessively, daydreaming how I'm going to save the children if this monster starts to go down.

Now, seven years later, Cathy is coming to Victoria for a visit because her husband is receiving an award for his research in fish fertility. She is bringing her boys. Nicholas is twelve, Anton seven. .

I open the door and Cathy and I hug, holding on for that extra thirty seconds to take in a breath together and let it go. Nicholas's hair is thick and so dark it's almost black, as are his eyes. Like his father, he's quiet yet fiercely present. Anton is fair-haired, hazel-eyed. His mouth hangs open because his muscles aren't strong enough to keep it closed. Cathy introduces Anton to me, says I knew him when he was a baby.

He says something that I don't quite catch because his speech is not fully defined.

"Can you say that again?" I ask, apologetic, and look from Anton to Cathy and back again.

"Is she hard of hearing, Mom?" he asks, slower this time and putting in more muscular effort so I understand. This kid is making fun of me as well as himself. It's as much a challenge as a moment of bonding.

"Oh, he's a charmer," says Cathy. "Aren't you, Anton?"

He smiles impishly and we all laugh.

He is a charmer, his wit even drier than his mother's.

The main floor of our house is upstairs and Anton expertly climbs the stairs backwards, on his bum. Cathy beams as he plays a mean jazz piece on the piano, trying to outdo his brother's earlier performance.

It happens to be Halloween, and after dinner Cathy and I walk Anton the vampire and my daughter the cat around to neighbouring houses. He walks unaided, a dip and twist to his movements, and tires after a short time. My daughter has been overexcited all day and she too tires quickly, happy to return home, where she and Anton greedily trade candy. Cathy tells me he will be hooked up to his stomach tube later that night in the hotel.

What strikes me most about Anton is the almost dismissive nonchalance he seems to have towards his condition. I wonder if this is for his mother's sake. Or if crashing for this child is just another form of flying.

EXHAUSTED, I HEAD UPSTAIRS AND check in on the three older kids, so uncomplicated in their sleep, so easy to love. Our seven-year-old still sleeps in our room, on a mattress on the floor pushed up against my side of the bed. I manoeuvre my way over her splayed limbs and slip in beside Bill.

FOUR MORE OF US

Bill Gaston

IT'S ODD THAT I REMEMBER only three of my children's births, because I was there for all four. Odder still is I don't remember the most recent. I wasn't drunk, I didn't faint, I didn't come running in too late from a poker game; it was nothing slapstick like that. I just don't remember.

LISE IS TWENTY NOW. I remember hers perfectly.

In trying to contribute this birth story, I recognize a feeling similar to one I had when Lise was born. It's a feeling of being a half-participant. In fact, maybe *half* is flattering myself. It's a feeling of being wanted and needed, yes, but also of being less than essential. (Maybe it's the reason I'm writing so formally and cautiously now, and not flinging the verve around.) It's a feeling of having only your hand—maybe only a finger—in the waterfall. You can feel its power but you're not drenched, unlike the mother, who's getting pounded, full force, hardly able to stand it, who's basically become an elemental force of nature herself.

In other words, I'm in a realm that's impossible for me to join. I'm fearful, cautiously happy, and a bit guilty to be here. Guilty? Well, she's over there screaming with a pain I'll never feel. By now she's also my best friend, but, for reasons of an extra chromosome, because of what we both enjoyed as equal partners (after a bit of tequila in Northampton, Massachusetts), she's screaming stiff on the bed there and I'm not. Capillaries burst in her cheeks as the pain peaks, and when it lessens she cries softly. That's the way it is — it's really not my fault — yet in the simplest sense it is. And I find that I want it to be, because at least then it connects me.

So though I'm just standing here watching, I'm suffering too, but mostly from abstractions, and since nothing's exploding in my face no one's about to feel sorry for me. But if they knew my mind, they would. I'm superstitious, deeply and maybe crazily so, and one thing I apparently believe is this: if you envision something bad, if you really picture it and suffer the image, it won't happen. So for eight months I'd been invoking possible nightmares, versions of the moment I first see our baby — a shock of too many limbs, or too few, or liverish organs throbbing outside the body, or inoperable facial bone defects, those genetic cul-de-sacs made manifest for all to see. Or a simpler one: a blue baby, dead. Alert to all the heart-melting stories out there, I'd been busy preparing for the worst. I'd also been revelling in stories of parents loving their Down babies, stories about cerebral palsy and genius. On a less tragic level, I was also steadying myself to experience life in an unpredictable new way, one there is no preparation for.

That's the stuff in my head, and here Dede's in labour. We're in Toronto East General and I know that for her this feels like defeat, though I'm secretly relieved. She's been in labour forty-five hours now, and the midwife who tried to grant her deep wish for a home birth has decided that a hospital has become necessary. Dede's strength is gone and she's prey to the bustling strangers, heartless machinery, and disinfectant; gone the perfect birth environment, the soft Beethoven, the gentle coos, worn blankets, and slightly creaky fan. Here in the hospital the head nurse, a Nurse Ratched truly, is telling our midwife (who's an archaic threat to her honour and livelihood) to shut up and stay out of the way. Dede is weak and whimpering, depressed now, and though I am but a petrified stick man, I do my best to be soothing and to sound honest as I suggest that every new kink in her carefully choreographed birth plan is really for the best. As when we learn that we can't wait any longer and the baby must be induced. As when Dede nods for the last-ditch epidural. Our doctor, Joe, a friend, has been here before and does a better job of it than me in convincing her that all is still fine. Willing fluidity to my arm, I rub her back the way we learned in class, and I try to adjust to Dede's *lower, harder, stop, where's your hand*, knowing I fail her by lacking a hand that knows her wants implicitly. At times, almost miraculously, we find each other's eyes, and some humour, and the best-friend part of things, and there's love rather than fear and pain—but now things kick in and go crazy. I'll go to my grave humbled by the power of this phrase: *she's going into transition.*

There begins a timeless chaos of hunched screaming, where no moment is anything other than emergency. Now our baby does fly out, at a speed hard to see and in a way that jostles time, that breaks your mind. The baby looks very small. Someone says, "It's a girl." I'm suddenly crying in big, gobby breaths, which is a surprise since I haven't cried in twenty or thirty years, and I can't stop sobbing as a nurse hauls the little bundle up onto Dede, whose face is indescribable with a joy that's quiet and knowing. My sobs have eased off to snivels and some laughing as I'm handed scissors and I cut a ridiculously blue cord the consistency of steak sinew. The blood flows almost black from the cut I make.

Lise (we don't name her for a few more days, but she's always been Lise) teaches me a few things right off the top. Her head is shaped like a thick banana, and I am shocked by this despite having learned about the skull's passage through the pelvis and all the rest. But I know from her piercing look that she is not only mentally fine but intellectually formidable. I know she can only focus within a foot, and Dede's face and mine are exactly that away from hers as we three intensely check each other out. We hardly breathe. Lise is wrestling with some drugs and with the exhaustion of what she's just done, and she has only a minute before a deep sleep sets in, but we learn a lot about each other in that time. And I can say without exaggeration that she hasn't really changed much at all since then. She can talk now, reads literary theory, in fact, but she was all there at less than a minute old. Maybe the biggest thing she taught me was that people arrive with emotional fecundity and a full being. Eye-to-eye with Lise in those first moments, I came to suspect that we arrive carrying a complete set of baggage, and that maybe they weren't her first moments at all.

CONNOR IS EIGHTEEN AND I remember lots.

Injured athletes watching from the sidelines are often heard to say it's *far* harder to watch than to play. That's right, I suppose I'm equating giving birth to *playing*. And, that's right, I'm saying it's harder watching. Okay, fine, every mother reading this has dismissed me as a deluded pig, but let's just say it's *possible* that I had the tougher time. As a delivering mother you can *do* stuff.

In fact you are doing so much stuff you are overwhelmed and, from the looks of it, thinking isn't even required. Watching— aside from the back rubbing and hand squeezing and those other ploys intended to keep the man distracted—there's nothing that Western culture allows a man to do with nine months of pent-up worry and testosteronic adrenalin. *At childbirth, we would love to explode.* So she suffers physically, I suffer mentally. Which is worse? I don't think I'm trying to be funny or confrontational when I say I don't know.

Dede is abundantly swollen again and it's her due date. Lise, nearly two, is home enjoying maybe her first babysitter, and we are in downtown Halifax for a film and a modest dinner out because it's the last time in a while when this might happen. Dede passes on restaurant food, opting for constant snacks from her treat bag, easily keeping her stomach, which has been shoved up into her throat and squeezed to the size of a lemon, full. I eat a Harvey's burger in the car on the way home to Hatchett Lake, have sympathy indigestion in bed that night, and then Dede's labour starts. I remember her labouring at home, out on the deck in a weak January sun, hanging on to a rail, squatting to let gravity do some of the work.

By mid-morning Dede's blood pressure is iffy, and the midwife decides we live a bit too far from Halifax General and we'd best go in. Once again Dede's wish for a home birth is quashed. In we drive, Dede sad, me not really.

As I am about to witness a second birth, it will help explain my state of mind if I describe Dede's relationship with the medical establishment.

Her desire for a home birth issued from a belief that birth is a natural, not medical, event. She also owned a genuine distrust of Western medicine. For one thing, she felt the wisdom of older, gentler ways. For another, her grandfather had died quickly of cancer, aged thirty-two, after taking massive X-ray "treatments" for acne. For yet another, as a professional ballet dancer and Buddhist, Dede was an astute student of both the mind and the body. I considered myself a holistic type too, but when we met, Dede had me beat by a mile. She knew her herbals and homeopathics; I was a dabbler. When she became pregnant, she educated herself on alternative and traditional childbirth, and was soon armed with stats about the evils of cow's milk, hospitals as incubators for staph, the suspicious spike in C-sections in North America, the misguided episiotomy (for which she taught me the subtle "pleasures" of perineal massage).

My position on Dede's position as we drive in from Hatchett Lake? That establishment medicine might mash you under its callous boot, but at least you'll crawl out alive. But because Dede is the pregnant one here, what she says goes.

So for a second time we arrive at a hospital, Dede wounded by it and feeling vulnerable. I am publicly saddened because she needs me to match her mood, but once more I'm secretly relieved. I'm suffering enough already. Sure, we've had one healthy birth, so I know it's possible. But superstition's logic hisses at me that we've dodged a bullet, teased fate, and are doubly overdue for tragedy.

Once more we get set up, our midwife introduces herself to suspicious nurses, and I commence rubbing Dede's back and trying to say the right things. Why does *I love you so much*, whispered sincerely in her ear during a rough spot, sound so hollow? Probably because, though I do feel it, it's what I'm supposed to say.

Things get heavy, things get fast. Dilated four centimetres, five centimetres. She screams, she shits, the nurse actually tells her, "You don't have to be so loud." The midwife, braver than me and doing my job, tells Dede to breathe with the pain and to be as expressive as she likes. At this point the nurse more or less shoulders the midwife out of the way and says that one person in the way is enough, meaning me, and the midwife is made to stand over near the wall.

I'm freaked out, praying, hanging on. The doctor has made her arrogant appearance, late, transition having come and gone. The baby is coming. Dede can't not push, she's bellowing, making the rhino noises I haven't heard for two years. Now she's allowed to push; she yells at the baby to *get out*. When the head appears, the doctor twists almost on her side and her hands go in and do something expert and acrobatic. *Something's different*, the voice hisses in my head. The doctor's urgency makes everything still, and all my nightmares come true when she says in soft singsong: "Cord, around, the neck…"

I almost die, maybe I do die, and she continues the same song: "Cord, slips off, easily…"

And now the baby shoots out and I'm seeing its beautiful body, bigger than Lise's, healthy, and once again I'm sobbing robustly while someone calls, "It's a boy!" and even though I truly never had a wish for anything but health, at hearing it's a boy I feel an extra surge, and to this day I wonder if this was because I was a man with a son or a father with one of each.

Snivelling, cutting another cord, I notice that one of our boy's ears is flat on top. The other is round, normal. So he's sort of deformed. I understand it means absolutely nothing—what's a deformed ear in the face of what could have been? You grow hair over a deformed ear. You wear hats.

And here it is, the intense, hushed, loving curiosity of three heads together, the baby's clear eyes (he wasn't yet Connor but had always been Connor) checking out the room, these faces. He knows he's safe. He's already looking beyond his parents a bit. He radiates an odd confidence and what seems like wisdom, but also an irony. Like Lise, he doesn't cry right away. Unlike Lise, he isn't drugged and doesn't need to sleep yet. Like Lise, he teaches me things. He is so different from his big sister and his mother and me, I learn that we all arrive deeply unique. I also learn from him that, no matter how close people get, and try to get, we will always be alone.

EARLIER, I AGREED TO SOME things Dede asked of me. I'm to help guard against such things as scalpels near her perineum, silver nitrate in eyes, and after the birth I'm to be with the baby at all times when they whisk him off to wash and weigh and clean up that first tarry black poop and then dress him in blue. Dede is a far more assertive person than I am. Following on the heels of a nearly angry nurse carrying Connor, I understand that in insisting I be present I am basically insulting her, accusing her of incompetence, cruelty, perhaps losing the baby altogether. I'm tempted to try to make it right, to suck up to her and say something like, *Sorry about this, but the wife, you know, she's a bit, well, let's just say I'm doing this for her.* Or maybe try the risqué joke that nurses lost our first one. But I keep quiet and follow her as she starts her chores. She lets me help with the weighing, washing, wrapping. I'm intensely curious about the smallest details of this child and, truth be told, the last thing I want to do is let him out of my sight.

VAUGHN IS FIFTEEN. HOW can I forget?

In our third attempt at a home birth we have a false alarm. Thinking labour has begun, our midwife drives all the way from Nova Scotia. A week later, when real labour comes on fast, she tells us over the phone that she wouldn't make it in time. So to Fredericton General we go.

This birth was marked by Dede's mother being in attendance. She'd always wanted to witness one, and she had travelled up from Virginia to do so. This all sounded understandable, even admirable to me, except that Millicent Crane was my *mother-in-law*. Though we like each other now, at the time we had a comedically clichéd in-law relationship. Dede naively thought that her being there was cool. Well, to put the situation succinctly, Dede was a highly trained ballet dancer, and her mother a dance mother and aesthetic freak whose single comment about hair or posture could ignite in the daughter a paralytic frenzy.

So here we are in the hospital for a third failed time, Dede's mother looking over my shoulder. I'm not as petrified this time, I find. For one, it's the middle of the day and I'm riding a good sleep. For another, after two births most of my nerve endings that register fear have been scraped dead (ask survivors of the Battle of Britain, skydivers, mail carriers in a neighbourhood of Dobermans: you remain afraid for only so long). But I knew that if I let down my guard, if I made the mistake of telling myself something like "birth is a natural, not a medical situation" or, most dangerous of all, "birth should be a joyous occasion," the birth would flip into nightmare and I would have caused it.

Dede is doubly irritable this time as I rub her back that way, this way, no that way, *that way*. There's a persistent shrillness to her voice, and now when her mother asks if she can do anything, Dede lashes out, and in her voice I hear it: not just the child, but the child getting revenge.

My sense is that Dede's glad I'm standing between the two of them. I think her mother is glad too, especially once her daughter gets to howling and grunting. Is she even louder this time? Is this also a bit of revenge? Dede's mother, whose experience of birthing her three children was being put to sleep and waking up the next day with a new, washed babe in arms, is also from the school of June Cleaver aesthetics — no unrehearsed noises, no hair out of place, no exploded capillary showing through one's makeup. Added to the scenario (more revenge?) is Dede's experiment with a new delivery position. She's come to understand that the woman-on-her-back method works against gravity, turning the tailbone's curve into a painful speedbump, favouring only the pediatrician, who could loom paternalistically above. Dede has options this time. She eschews the rice-paddy squat, considers the side pose but lacks the right pillows, and opts in the end for on-all-fours. "I'm going hands and knees," she calmly tells me between rhino calls, and she does.

So Dede's on all fours, rhino-ing all the more, her mother edging towards the hallway, maybe the parking lot, and here is maybe my starkest memory of all four births. Now Vaughn (not yet named, but always Vaughn) is still a contrary kid, and he had decided to come out transverse (called "back labour," it's maybe why Dede chose all fours). In any case, here I am, as directed by the doctor, ready to support the baby's head, which will emerge but stall there, while he works the shoulder free.

My hands are loosely cupped as if to catch a coconut. Now the baby's crowning, that strange bluish colour with the powder-white of vernix, then crowning more, and now here's a whole head — *pop*, a head in my hands — a head with a face, a face with eyes looking at me. I'm standing at Dede's side, and here's this little head sticking out of what seems to be her bum, and the head's eyes are open and looking around, and I'm stooped to get my own face in close and our eyes lock, and I swear the baby smiles *mischievously*, this baby who is either a boy or a girl, but that part doesn't matter at all, because I can see the capricious, sparky being whose head is in my hands and whose face is so entirely his/her own. This person is not only right into the adventure, this person already wants to win.

"Hi," I say.

The baby's eyes flit here, there, everywhere with speed, trying to take in the game whose rules he/she wants to learn; I can see the child's excitement from the wild ride it's just had, and it knows more is coming; and I can tell that this baby is mostly listening, with antennae I can't see, electric with hungry sense. The eyes want to see everything and they blink hard, bothered by the light, and I can't remember who called for the curtains to be closed but I think it was me.

So I get to know Vaughn quite well, even before I know if he's male or female. Capricious, bright, funny, lonely—nothing I saw in these first moments has changed.

Though I knew that this child was smart and healthy, I didn't cry yet. My sobbing, and his crying, didn't start until he flew out.

LILLI IS NINE NOW, and maybe the stork brought her.

The weird thing is, Dede has had to help me with this one. I sit and think but can't recall, for instance, what time we drove to the hospital.

"You don't remember?" she asks.

"Not a clue." Not even if it was day or night.

"You don't remember how calm it was in the streets? That it was the middle of the night?"

"No." Though now I start to, I start to. And what I start to remember most is the *feeling* of this fourth birth, my feeling. Basically, there was no panic. Essentially, I wasn't afraid.

Dede keeps asking. "And how the hospital was deserted? There was no one in the halls at all? But we knew where to go, and just went to the delivery area? You were carrying my big blue ball?"

It sort of starts coming back. Yes, I do remember the vacant hallways. And how non-nervous we both were. Child number four. I think I recall jokes about that Monty Python flick, the baby falling out into a bucket while Mother does the dishes. I recall that we had no midwife this time because we decided we didn't really need one, we both knew all the lore now. I remember too that Fredericton General was no failure this time but our choice. A kind of shrug, no big deal. It was just easier and safer, and we both knew how to stand up for the stuff that was worth standing up for—no silver nitrate, minimal fetal heart-monitor strips, some laughing gas taken orally. And it seems the nurses and doctors respected our wishes now, these two old pros who knew how it all worked. We'd simply gotten more casual, had learned that birth isn't really a medical event but that hospitals had a pretty good set-up for it. Use it, then lose it, in and out fast. Dede has always loved her own bed. With Vaughn's birth she'd put a roast in the oven before going to the hospital, and after having Vaughn—and after I signed release and waiver forms under the disapproving gazes of doctors and staff—Dede and Vaughn and I were home before the roast was done. This time, child number four, maybe we'd just head home and cut the cord there.

Yes, and I do recall now that walk through the hallway and the feeling of being Mom and Pop Childbirth, a holding-hands feeling, a quiet but deep love and a tired knowledge that we had some work ahead of us but that there would be some vast reward at the end of it, so vast you couldn't really hang a name or even a feeling on it. One thing I'd learned, from Vaughn, was that each child brought with it a completely different kind of love, as original as the child itself.

"Lilli had the most perfect eyebrows."

"Really?"

"You don't remember?"

"How did you deliver Lilli?" Because I have no image, none at all.

"On my side. My right side." She hesitates. "You don't remember?"

"Sort of." But I don't. It's gone.

"Don't you remember catching her?"

"I caught her?"

"She was the first one you actually caught, by yourself."

Funny. It's significant, maybe, that Lilli was the only one I caught. Even today we're physical all the time. We push, we tussle, she demands to be carried, and even if we're mad at each other she'll be right up on my lap, because we're most comfortable together when we're touching. Even though she's way too big now, when I'm lying prone in my La-Z-Boy she'll crawl up and lie on me like I'm a bed. She never asks permission and doesn't need it. It's pretty much automatic. Lise, well, occasionally she'll walk into my semi-formal hug. As for the boys, physical contact is long gone, and when I remember being allowed by them to carry, wrestle, stroke, and hand-hold in the mall, I could almost cry. These days, their only physical connection to me is the wondering, at a deeply ape or perhaps Freudian level, whether they could topple me and get a foot on my neck.

But I remember Lise's eyes, and Connor's expression, and Vaughn's face so clearly. And I picture cutting all those cords, though they all looked the same — the pulsing, the bright silver-blue, and that spurt of deepest red-black blood.

I'm starting to catch on why I don't remember Lilli's. Likely I remember my other three, as I do my father's death, because of the panic. There's something about stark emergency that etches stone. With Lilli I was relaxed. I had finally relaxed. I do believe I maybe even enjoyed myself.

"I didn't cry with Lilli, did I?"

"No."

But I'm sad for having so very few memories of Lilli coming into the world, only nine years ago. What she's taught me is that to relax is also somehow to go to sleep. She tells me that, during birth, if the emotions are as high as the stakes, then your memories resemble the screaming sitcoms you've seen, and all the clichés are true.

It also seems true that birth can be as electric and moving an event as death, where both time and light become something else. The difference with birth, of course, is that it has brought another of us. After the explosion you stand in the fold, three touching heads breathing short, almost-held breaths, and it feels and sounds and smells like nothing else. For the baby, there's no notion yet of Other, so she's only content to include you in her sense of herself. To her, the love must feel like the most natural part of it. Hushed, and so gentle as to be elegant, it feels like the three of you aren't touching ground. I've experienced this trinity of heads with all four of my children, and sadly I can recall only three of them. But it's something you can't quite recapture in memory anyway, or in words either.

MY PERFECT BIRTH

Stephanie Nolen

FOR ABOUT FORTY PERFECT minutes, I had the birth I wanted: the bright gold of autumn sunlight streamed in the open windows, the music of a Ugandan drum band filled the kitchen, and lentil soup—the most practical thing my best friend, Marney, could think to make for a birth—bubbled on the stove. In between contractions, I lolled in my big blue birth tub in the middle of the kitchen floor, sucking on an orange Popsicle and making jokes to Marney and my sister Amy. When the contractions came, I rolled on to my knees and my partner, Meril, or our doula, Jennifer, cradled my head on the edge of the pool, and I gave the pain a voice—a deep, guttural sound that was somewhere between a hum and a groan. "Ride it out—you can do it," Jennifer would say softly, and the wave of pain would crest and fall away. Then I'd reach for the Popsicle and resume the conversation.

It wasn't quite Ina May Gaskin. I'd read and reread Ina May during my pregnancy: a pioneering midwife who revived the art in the United States in the 1960s, Ina May supervised thousands of home births on a commune in Tennessee. Her book *Spiritual*

Midwifery is part philosophical tract, part medical textbook, and part compendium of dozens of birth stories. Sometimes she irritated me — Ina May won't let labouring women use the word "contraction" and insists on calling them "rushes." The book is full of goofy testimonials from women who talk about "smooching with my honey when the rushes were coming on so that we were all feeling groovy." But births with Ina May are celebrations — the stories in the book are of calm and safe and peaceful births, where the labouring women are beautiful and powerful. That was the birth I wanted.

And I had come a long way to have it: I live in South Africa, the country that has the highest rate of Caesarean sections in the world for hospital births — 80 percent. The majority of South African women are poor, black women who give birth at home or in rural clinics with limited medical intervention. But in Johannesburg, every single woman I knew had given birth in a hospital and had had a C-section — one of them because her obstetrician wanted to holiday in Mauritius on her due date, another because her doctor thought she "might have some tearing." I began the hunt just hours after I found out I was pregnant, and quickly discovered that there wasn't a single midwife who would support me through a home birth. Most of them had never heard of Ina May, and if they had, they thought she was a crackpot. And so, on the last possible day I was allowed to fly, I wedged my belly into a 747 seat and headed for Canada — to Kingston, Ontario, where we had a couple of friends who told us of a wonderful midwifery practice that did home births every day.

In Kingston, I came into the care of a warm and lovely midwife named Jane. We rented a house with a light-filled kitchen and had a birth pool shipped up from Toronto. A week after my due date — when I had taken to sleeping like a horse, standing and leaning on

my forearms, because the pain in my hips was so excruciating—
I finally felt what I was sure were contractions. With a flutter of
excitement deep in my belly, I sat at the kitchen table in the early
morning trying to read the Sunday *New York Times* (aware that this
might be the last moment for thirty years that I would have time
on a Sunday to read it all the way through), and then we began the
phone calls: to my sister, to tell her to get on a train from Ottawa;
to my in-laws in Cape Breton, so they could begin their anxious
pacing; to my best friend, so she could start the soup.

And, of course, to the midwives. First I called Jane. Her voice
mail said she was off-duty for the weekend, a calamity I had been
braced for. So I called her backup midwife: the voice mail said
she'd been at a birth all night and gave another name and number.
I could no longer talk through the contractions, so I handed the
phone to Meril and he started to work his way through the roster:
up all night at a birth, said message after message. The last of the
practice's eight midwives said in a recording, "I've been up for two
days at a birth. If you can't find a midwife, go to the hospital."

"Go to the hospital?" I wailed to Meril. "We just flew seven
thousand kilometres to have a home birth!"

It was, we later learned, the first time in the ten-year history of
the midwifery practice that this had ever happened: the midwives
caught eight babies in forty-eight hours that weekend, and mine,
alas, was last in line. The midwives were wrung out and off duty.
Now my excitement had turned to a sharp and rancorous anxiety.

Eventually one of the midwives, Heather, called me back.
I told her I was in labour and she said, wearily, that, given that
this was my first baby, it would likely be about seventeen hours
before I was ready to deliver—to try to sleep (Sleep!) and call
her back later. I put the phone down. Anxiety turned to panic:
do this for seventeen more hours? Seventeen?

Right about then Jennifer the doula showed up. Jennifer, veteran of more than fifty births, took one look at me — on my hands and knees on the mattress we'd laid on the living room floor while the birth tub warmed — and had Meril call the midwife back to tell her it wasn't going to be seventeen hours.

I know in retrospect that a lot of things began to happen around then, although I recall them only in a haze. My sister and my best friend bustled in; I started to vomit between contractions; Heather the midwife arrived and, I gather, had a look at my cervix (one might think I would recall more about that, but I remember only the shiny green surface of the big inflated ball I was leaning on); and I fell in love with Jennifer, who seemed the only person in the world who understood how I was feeling.

And then, at last, the pool was full and warm and I could get in it. The pain immediately subsided, and I became once again a person who could cope.

"Turn up the stereo," I said. "And do we still have any potato salad?"

In the background I was vaguely aware of the midwife rustling around, but I knew that I had every possible supply needed for this home birth neatly arranged on the counter. (Twelve facecloths: check. Eight receiving blankets: check. Two trash bags: check. Mirror: check. Flashlight: check.) I was peaceful in the water, comfortable, and even able to be excited, rather than nervous, about what was to come.

And then I rolled onto my knees during one of those contractions and felt the oddest *pop!* and a funny sort of shifting inside. It was nothing like the moment of waters breaking I'd read about, and most likely no one would have noticed it had happened, except that Meril was fussing behind me about the temperature of the pool, and he saw an inky swirl pour from between my legs, quickly dissipating in the tub. He waved the midwife over and, in an instant, the peaceful joy of my Ina May Gaskin home birth fell away.

"Stephanie, that was your water breaking, and there seems to be meconium—a lot of meconium," Heather said in her midwife voice: calm, respectful, alarmed. "That means..."

I knew what it meant. Baby poo in the amniotic sac is a sign of possible fetal distress. In a second my hippie mama vibe vanished and I became the old me. I could see that Meril, my sister, and Marney all recognized this person, although they were a bit astonished to see her reappear at this moment.

"It means we go to the hospital," I said. "Just run through for me what the risks are of staying here."

Heather began to talk about what distress could mean, how she couldn't monitor me properly in the tub.

"Right," I said. "Amy, can you get my suitcase, it's in the hall upstairs. Meril, please get me some clothes. Someone turn off the stove. Meril, don't forget my wallet—my health card's in it."

I issued instructions and I bit back hard on my disappointment. I had dreamed of this home birth, but I would not insist on staying at home if there was any hint that the baby or I needed attention that could be had only at the hospital. The words of a friend in Jo'burg echoed in my head: "You're having a baby, not a birth."

But I was scared. I had had very little fear as I approached the birth—in part, perhaps, because my pregnancy had been so truly horrendous that it was difficult to believe anything could be worse—but also because, in my work as a journalist in Africa, I'd seen many women giving birth. I'd seen them lean on trees, on each other, on their hands and knees in bare-bones labour wards, and it gave me a visceral knowledge that I too could do this.

Now, though, as I listened to the suddenly somber houseful of people rushing to prepare for the hospital transfer, my confidence drained away. I could do this in the pool, with the people I loved around me. But in a hospital, separated from all of them except Meril and the doula? (Idiotic hospital rules said a woman could bring only two people with her into the delivery room.) I was not at all sure that I could do that. The pain seemed suddenly twice as fierce, and the next time I rolled to my knees I heard a scream — a thin, high-pitched scream — come from my throat, a noise unlike anything I'd ever made before.

When the next gap came, I hauled myself to my feet and pulled on a T-shirt and pajama bottoms. Next gap, down the hall. Next gap, front steps. Jennifer's minivan was parked out front, its two side doors and rear hatch all open. I climbed in the nearest door, got one knee up on a seat, fell to my elbows on the floor, and waited. Nothing happened. I looked up. Meril was at one side door, Jennifer at the other, Marney at the back, all of them staring at me.

"Are you going to stay like that?" they asked in a chorus.

"What the fuck does it look like?" I snarled, asking myself how I had ever collected such a bunch of blockheads to attend my birth.

They scurried into the car and we began to move. Moments later I had to vomit again, and I motioned frantically to Meril for the bowl. He'd forgotten it. There was nothing, it turned out, in the car for me to vomit into. But I wasn't going to throw up in Jennifer's car: I loved Jennifer. She alone understood me. I had to protect her upholstery. I felt my cheeks pouch out, and then farther out. I was Satchmo, mouth bulging as the car inched through crowds of revellers in the Kingston streets. (It was Homecoming Weekend, and every drunken Queen's student was apparently standing in the road between me and the hospital.)

When at last we pulled up at the Emergency Room doors, I backed down out of the car into a wheelchair and spit the vomit somewhere. I took my glasses off and handed them to Jennifer: if I had to be in a hospital, I wanted to see as little of it as possible. I would not put my glasses on again until there was a baby in my arms.

That, in the end, was rather sooner than anyone expected. But I was still working on the seventeen hours premise. I got down on my hands and knees in the delivery room, the chilly hospital tile instantly making my knees throb, and tried to think how I was going to endure this pain. Jennifer sat cross-legged in front of me, her voice the one constant in my world: sometimes she said gentle things about riding the wave, and sometimes she said, "That hurts like hell, hey? God, that hurts." Somehow she always knew which I needed. My sister and Marney had snuck past the nursing staff to join us, and now everyone was with me, but I could hear only Jennifer.

Having given up all dreams of my perfect birth, I was now demanding an epidural; if I couldn't be in my pool, in my kitchen, and I had to be on the vicious cold floor, then I wanted drugs, and to hell with Ina May. Jennifer tried gently to explain that it could be a long time before they found an anesthetist on a Sunday afternoon, and in the meantime, Heather the midwife proffered nitrous oxide. When the next contraction came, she held a black mask over my face and instructed me to breathe. But this was the wrong pain management technique to offer a war correspondent: the mask was black and rubber and smelled vile, and suddenly I was back in Baghdad, back in Gaza, back in a bomb shelter. I swatted it furiously off my face. Heather backed away. She had not slept in days; she went off in search of food and asked Anita (another midwife from the practice, who was in the hospital to check on a new mother) to substitute briefly. I couldn't see Anita without my glasses and on my knees, but I grunted consent when she said she wanted a look at my cervix.

"Huh," she said. "Nine centimetres."

I started to feel an intense sort of pressure, something I couldn't control. A few minutes later Anita looked over at me from across the room and asked, incredulous, "Are you pushing?"

"Uh, I don't think so?" I said. I'd been in active labour just three hours. It would be seventeen, Heather had said. So I couldn't be pushing.

I would learn later that through all of this there had been a current of drama to which I was largely oblivious. The midwives had been trying in various ways to position a monitor that would pick up the baby's heartbeat, without success, and now Anita insisted that I get up on the bed briefly while they had an obstetrician insert a monitor through my cervix and attach it to my baby's head. Meril had started to read to me about this procedure from one of my towering stack of birth books a few days earlier, and I cut him off. "That's horrible," I said. "That's not going to happen to us." And now I was being instructed to lie perfectly still through a contraction that felt like being threaded through a laundry mangle while an obstetrical resident put a wire through my cervix and poked it into my baby's scalp.

When it was done, after a minute or two, they let me get back down on the floor. I didn't notice the increasing alarm with which everyone was looking at the monitor screen: the baby's heart rate was falling by half with each contraction.

Anita came over and told me, none too gently, that I was going to have to get on the bed. I could still be on my knees; they would raise the head of the bed and let gravity help. By now I was outright pushing: puffing those cheeks back out and straining with each contraction. Soon Anita was back, even more brusque. I couldn't stay on my knees, she said, but she had a squat bar, so I could squat in the bed, holding myself up with the bar. Two pushes like that and I heard Heather say to her, "It looks like we're going to have to do McRoberts."

The McRoberts position, I can now tell you, involves having the labouring woman lie on her back, with someone holding each knee in the air and another supporting her back, and at each contraction folding her up, using the same physical principle used to get the last glob out of a tube of toothpaste. I'd barely spoken since we arrived at the hospital, but now — as Marney held my head, Jennifer held one of my hands and Meril the other, Heather and Anita each hauled one of my knees up near my ears — I choked out, "I thought I just flew seven thousand kilometres to give birth with a midwife so I didn't end up on my goddamn back with my knees in my ears." No one replied.

The baby's heart rate was dropping more dramatically with each contraction, and — I learned later — Anita was battling with the obstetrical staff (who could follow the monitor on a second screen out at the nursing station) to maintain control over the birth and stave off medical intervention. She had a hunch that the baby was fine, heart rate notwithstanding, but she couldn't keep me in midwifery care for very long.

"You need to have this baby in two contractions," she said to me.

I was by this point far inside myself, eyes sealed closed. I was thinking about canoe trips, about long, hot portages when the canoe presses down like an iron bit into my shoulders and salty sweat stings in the corner of my eyes and blackflies needle my legs and I can't swat them and it feels with each step like my calves and cheeks are being drilled down into the path and I'm certain, certain, that I won't ever see the glimmer of water through the trees ahead—and how, in the end, the lake is always there, and I can stop, and there is that moment of merciful freedom when I summon the last strength in my arms to push the canoe up and off my shoulders and the cool air hits my face. There's always the lake, if I can just keep walking with that canoe on my shoulders.

That's where I was.

And now this woman—this woman I couldn't even see—was telling me I had to have a baby in two contractions. A baby?

At some level I knew the situation was becoming increasingly urgent and that I had to do what she said. So I pulled from the soles of my feet and the top of my head, channelling all the strength I could into the fiery ache in the middle of my body, and pushed.

And then Anita said, "Here's the head. Do you want to feel the head?"

I ignored her. I let someone manoeuvre my hand between my legs, but felt nothing.

Then Anita spoke again.

I should tell you here that in the last weeks of my pregnancy, I lumbered to the midwives' office and borrowed every birth book in their library. I was drawn in particular to the old books, their covers held on by yellowing Scotch Tape, and I became enamoured with the French obstetrician Michel Odent, who in the 1970s remade the way women gave birth at Pithiviers Hospital in France. His book, *Birth Reborn*, had pages filled with photos of gorgeous women, their faces raw emotion, standing up and leaning against a lover or the good doctor himself, their hands reaching down to catch the baby sliding from their bodies. This was what I imagined, reaching down in my birth pool to catch the baby myself as I pushed it into the world. I wrote it into my birth plan.

But now Anita said, "Stephanie, do you want to catch your baby?" And I felt a flash of rage.

"For chrissake," I spat out. "There are five other people around this fucking bed. Is there no one else who can catch the fucking baby? I'm a little busy."

And I pushed. I heard Marney start to cry, saying, "I can see the head!" And I heard Meril start to give great, laughing sobs. And I pushed again, and saw Anita reaching and fumbling, and then this enormous slimy creature with long, spidery limbs was lying on my suddenly slack belly.

Jennifer plonked my glasses back on my nose and supported my shoulders. I looked down, hunting in the tangle of limbs and cord and ooze for a face. There were little blue eyes, the colour of my own, and I felt sure, as those eyes met mine, that we had the same baffled expression on our faces.

Meril cut the umbilical cord. The obstetrical people, who were now piling into the room, whisked the baby off my belly.

"What is it?" I asked, as I felt the sudden absence of him.

No one knew what I meant at first, and finally — many minutes after his birth — someone said to me, "A boy. He's a boy."

The obstetrical residents began to poke and prod him, although it was clear from his glossy pink skin and his startled wailing that there was nothing wrong with him at all; just as Anita had thought, neither the meconium nor the dipping heartbeat had meant distress. I leaned back and caught my breath, and when I could focus my eyes, noticed they were messing about with my baby.

"Give him back," I said loudly. And then I yelled: "GIVE ME BACK MY DAMN BABY."

Startled, the doctors stepped back from their work table, and Meril scooped up the baby and handed him back to me. I saw the midwives exchange a smile.

He was gorgeous, our boy. He was looking all around, bemused. I wanted him near me, but I didn't feel—not yet— that wave of maddened love I'd read about. Instead, all I could think about, all I could talk about, was the fact that I was no longer pregnant. Only ten minutes after his birth—long before the midwife had begun to stitch up my shredded perineum with several packs of sutures—I felt like myself again for the first time in forty-one weeks. I felt gloriously normal.

We have no good pictures of this birth because my sister the med student was put in charge of the camera. I have many photos that could illustrate an edition of *Advanced Obstetrics*, images where you can see up through my vagina to my tonsils, but none that contain my face. But I remember being both exhausted and filled by a huge surge of adrenalin, I remember plowing into the monstrous crate of snacks Marney had brought (she was prepared for a three-day labour), I remember laughing while she wrapped her arms around me and told me how amazing I was. I remember thinking, *Damn right*. I remember saying to Meril, "Did you see what I just did?" I was in breathless awe of myself.

Soon I was stitched and showered, and I had managed, after considerable effort, to pee, which meant the midwives were willing to discharge me, not quite three hours after we arrived at the hospital. My boy had had a first nurse, latching on happily, and Meril and I dressed him in the tiny outfit I had washed over and over again to make it soft.

We snapped the little car seat into Jennifer's van and went home, where the water in the birth tub was barely cool, and there was still potato salad. I settled my baby on my shoulder, picked up a plate with a big piece of pie, and climbed the stairs to our bed, to settle in and begin a lifetime of being mesmerized by his face.

MOON WOMAN

Afua Cooper

THE DOCTOR SUGGESTED I TAKE a drug to speed up the labour. It was 2:00 p.m. on July 20, 1981, and I had been in labour since 5:00 a.m. the day before. Thirty-three hours of attempting to birth a child. My first child. I was tired, but not exhausted. I was young and in great physical shape: the many years of yoga had paid off. The nurse attending to me agreed that I should take the medication. My partner, Patrick, also agreed. Everyone felt that the labour had gone on for too long.

"The child is not ready," I said to them.

I HAD ARRIVED IN CANADA eight months earlier. I had just turned twenty-three, and I was already two months pregnant. For me, pregnancy was a romantic affair. A beautiful adventure. I felt like a moon woman, or a fecund earth mother and goddess, bringing new life to the world.

In Jamaica, where I had come from, most people gave birth in the hospital. If labour came on too quickly then some women ended up having their children at home, as my mother did with my younger sister. She sent for my grandmother, who delivered the child.

Then there was the great institution of the district nurse. This health professional worked mainly in the rural areas. She referred the cases she could not deal with to a clinic or hospital. She was also a midwife, and women who did not want to have hospital births arranged with the district nurse to deliver their children at home. The district nurse in the area where I grew up wore a brown uniform and starched cotton headgear. She also drove a car.

In Jamaica, giving birth and having a child was a natural thing. People loved children and saw them as gifts from God. People pitied women who did not have children. It was felt that a household was especially blessed if children were present. The best noise in a house, the elders would say, is the sound of a baby or children playing.

I grew up with children around me. My elder sisters, cousins, and neighbours had babies, and I learnt how to look after them, bathe them, feed them, sing to them, play with them. I helped to raise them. A woman had a strong support system to help her and the child, and she could therefore continue with her job and career. Children were a natural part of life, in the same way as eating and breathing. Giving birth was one of the things that women did—because they were women. And only they could do it.

In Canada, I detected that people did not like children. They tolerated them. Moreover, people also seemed to want everything to be in place before they had children—they had to have a house, with the mortgage almost paid for, to be ensconced in their careers and have lumps of money in the bank. Getting pregnant and having a child was another thing they placed on a to-do list and then ticked off once it was accomplished.

I also realized that in Canada, and North America in general, there was a lot of intervention in the birth experience. The use of the epidural was quite normal. Using the knife to cut and widen the vagina and forceps to drag the baby from the birth canal was also standard procedure. For me, these practices were like medieval methods of torture.

I decided I was going to give birth as naturally as possible. I discovered Dr. Lamaze, and was attracted to the Lamaze method because I was already working with the breathing techniques through my practice of yoga. Painless childbirth, it was called. At the weekly Lamaze classes the main focus was on the breath. The breath was everything. "It is what will sustain you through your labour," our instructor, Susan, told us. She also insisted that we have objects to concentrate on. One should be so focused that when the labour pain pulses through the body, one rides it with the breath as one would ride a wave at the beach.

Every day I practised my Lamaze breathing. My object of focus was a star in the middle of a doily I had knitted. I pinned it to the wall and would concentrate on it while I breathed. Susan also encouraged us to go to the free public health prenatal course. We were taught baby care and postnatal exercises. Being in the company of other pregnant women eased some of the loneliness I felt as a new immigrant, and a pregnant one at that.

Susan also found me a doctor who agreed to do a natural birth. When I went for my first visit, we went over my birth plan—I made it clear that there was to be no intervention, no epidural or forceps, unless it was absolutely necessary. He did not think it necessary to do an ultrasound, although nowadays such a procedure is routine.

A part of me felt absolutely wonderful. I was in good health, my weight gain was fine, and I had no morning sickness. My diet was completely vegan. I went on long walks and was a macho meditator. Another part of me was homesick for Jamaica and experiencing severe culture shock. I grieved for the loss of those aspects of my culture that sustained and supported a woman and her new child.

On the morning of Sunday, July 19, 1981, at around 5:00 a.m., my water broke. I had just done two hours of yoga and was brimming with energy. I went to bed but could not sleep. Then I felt a gush of water between my legs. I knew I would not be sleeping anytime soon.

I prepared myself for the contractions. They began to come intermittently. I got up, made breakfast, ate, and forced myself to sleep. By 10:00 a.m. I was up, and I did the laundry and tidied the house while breathing through my contractions, which were coming every twelve minutes. I called my partner, who was working in the United States, and my relatives. I knew it was not time to go to the hospital: the contractions were slight and too far apart.

Sunday evening came. My partner arrived. The length of time between contractions lessened. I managed to get some sleep in between contractions. I was very excited. The phone rang. It was one of my cousins. He lived close by and his wife was as pregnant as I was. In fact, we used to joke about who would give birth first. My cousin was insisting that I go to the hospital. I told him the contractions were too far apart. If I were to go to the hospital, they would shove me into a labour room and leave me there until the contractions increased. But my cousin was fearful. For him, birth was a time of trepidation. I calmed his fears and he promised to call first thing in the morning.

Monday morning came and the contractions were coming more rapidly. My partner checked to see how much I was dilated.

Not much. My cousin came with his pregnant wife. I had now been in labour for twenty-four hours. All three insisted that I leave for the hospital. I told them it was still not time to go, but they would not take no for an answer. So I got my small suitcase and went to Queensway General Hospital. It was five in the morning. As I had predicted, I was taken to a labour room and left there. Around noon my doctor came, checked me, and said I was still not dilated enough. He was a little worried. He left for his office and said he would return soon. I drifted in and out of sleep. The doctor came back at around 4:00 p.m. He was not satisfied that the labour was progressing quickly enough. I was still not sufficiently dilated.

"If we go on like this," he said, "you will be giving birth on Tuesday." He suggested I take a drug to speed up the labour.

"The child's not ready," I told them, but finally the doctor talked me into it.

Immediately after being injected with the drug, contractions rolled on top of each other so rapidly, so fast, that I could not keep up with the breathing. Sweat poured from my body, and a pain like I had never before experienced in my life ripped through me. I cried.

My body convulsed as it danced a dance that women throughout the millennia have performed in order to bring new life into the world. The child that was descending was also doing its birth dance as forces beyond its control pushed it downwards, expelling it from my body. So much pain. I heard Susan telling me to focus on my breath. *Breathe with the contractions. Ride the waves.* Bile sprang into my mouth. I felt a bearing down. My body wanted to explode. My body, a woman's body, was stretching, straining, bruising, hurting, but at the same time engaging in an act of supreme love. The act of sex, the going up of a man's sexual organ, was responsible for this. Now the result of that love act was coming down nine months later. *Go on your journey, child. Embrace your journey. Good spirits travel with you.*

The nurses came, held my hands as I cried. Patrick rubbed my shoulders and my back. Looking back, I marvel at how I moved seamlessly between joy and pain and sorrow. One moment I was crying, but as the contraction passed I cracked jokes. That was how I was managing the labour. There were times when I was on top of it; other times, I succumbed to the pain. I had an overriding thought, and it was to be *present* and aware during my labour. I wanted this birth to be mine. Throughout it all I had good people around me and would not have made it had it not been for them. The nurses were wonderful and caring. Patrick was a rock.

At 6:15 p.m. I touched the area of my vagina and felt something like hair. The hair on the baby's head could be confused with the hair on the mother's body. I called Patrick, who called the nurse. She rushed in and looked. "Oh my God, the baby has crowned. I must call the doctor." She rushed out and another nurse rushed in and wheeled me into the delivery room. High drama. I was in pain and panting.

I breathed and focused on the point between my brows, the third eye. This spot, which is also known as the inner eye and the sixth chakra, is seen as the portal to higher consciousness. Focusing on the third eye allowed me to enter an inner space free from the physicality of the pain that was racking my body. I lay on my back, my legs propped up, a nurse at the foot of the bed, another nurse to the side. One nurse said she had called my doctor. He was at his office, close by on the West Mall. Another doctor rushed in. He was young. He held a knife-like instrument in his hand. He told the nurses to make me ready.

"Hold it," I said out loud. "Who are you?...My doctor and I agreed that he would only cut me if it was totally necessary." The doctor looked stunned.

"The baby is coming out," I said. "There is no need to cut me!" As if on cue, my doctor rushed in. I was never more relieved to see anyone. One nurse put the white outfit on him. Waves and waves of pain washed over me. I felt as if my body were in the middle of an ocean storm. I rode it out with concentrated breathing, yet I moaned and groaned. My partner held me on one side, a nurse gave support on the other side. I followed the doctor's instructions to "push and breathe." I felt an overwhelming urge to defecate. I said so to the nurse. She said it was normal and that it was the baby's weight bearing down on the rectum.

Then the baby's head slipped out to oohs and aahs in the room. Someone held a mirror for me to look. Its face was squished and red. The shoulders followed and next the entire body, accompanied by blood, water, and mucus.

"It is a boy," someone said, and the child and I cried simultaneously.

Everyone in the room then spoke at the same time. A cacophony of voices praising, giving thanks, congratulating. A nurse wrote on a pad.

"You gave birth at 7:35 p.m." she said to me.

Another wiped my private area. The doctor held the baby in his arms.

"Look, Patrick," he said. "He is perfect...perfect," and he raised the child up as if he were a prize.

The doctor passed the baby to me, and I held him and looked at him. He *was* perfect. A mat of black hair crowned his head. His complexion was the colour of wheat. I smiled broadly, the pain forgotten. His face was perfectly round, like a baby Buddha, and looking just as serene. My intuition about the sex of the baby had also been correct.

Still holding the baby, the doctor gave Patrick a scissors-like instrument to cut the umbilical cord.

"Are you sure?" he asked nervously.

"Yes, it is fine, go ahead," the doctor said.

Patrick cut the cord, and the bond that had united the baby with me for nine months was severed.

The doctor opened my legs and said, "Look, Patrick, look— no tear. She did not tear at all!" The nurses were also impressed. A nurse took the baby, cleaned him off, and wrapped him in white cotton clothing. Another nurse massaged and pressed on my abdomen, and the afterbirth slid out as my body went through its last spasm of pain.

The baby weighed five pounds, fifteen ounces, which they thought was a bit small for a full-term child. The doctor also thought he might be jaundiced because he looked yellow. So, in between nursings, he was placed under a lamp to normalize his colour. In retrospect I realized it was his normal complexion.

The time in the hospital was great. The nurses were kind and thoughtful. They taught me how to take a sitz bath to heal the trauma that the vagina and rectum had experienced during birth. They showed me how to make the baby latch onto the breast properly, how to bathe the baby, and how to care for the umbilical stump that was still attached to the navel area. They ensured that we ate our meals and got our rest. The babies stayed with their mothers during the daytime and were taken to the baby room at night. Mothers could, however, go to the baby room whenever they wanted to be with their child.

My doctor visited daily and gave me and the baby a clean bill of health. After three days I wanted to go home, but he insisted

I spend one full week. I look back at the time in the hospital as a nurturing time and one of rest. In those days women who went in to give birth were looked after very well. The week gave me and the other new mothers a time to gain and gather strength. In rural areas when I was growing up, the mother is bathed and fed and must stay inside the house for nine days after giving birth. Her only task is to nurse the baby. After nine days she and the child are allowed to sit on the porch, and can entertain visitors and well-wishers.

The nine days inside the house is a carry-over from African tradition and mirrors the nine months that the child is in the womb. It is a transition period in which both mother and child are introduced to the world that they must now inhabit. I also think it acts as a protection for the mother and child from malevolent spirits that roam the outside and would do harm to the child. Spirits love new babies and desire to carry them back to the world they have just left. My aunts told me that when they were growing up, the staying-in period was forty days instead of nine.

The name we chose for the baby would symbolize what we wished the child to become. So we named him Akil. It is Arabic for "intelligent and knowledgeable one."

MY SECOND BIRTH. It was February 1993. My circumstances had changed. I was no longer a new immigrant, unsure of myself in a strange and foreign country. By this time I had gained bachelor's and master's degrees, had worked in the fields of education and social work, had established myself as a poet and hoped to do the same as a scholar. I was also in my second long-term relationship. The relationship between Akil's father and me had dissolved, and I had married in 1991.

Shortly after my marriage I became pregnant but suffered

a miscarriage. Then I got pregnant again and went to term. At the time of the birth I was in a Ph.D. program at the University of Toronto and was also working as a teaching assistant. My life revolved around the university. I loved my studies. I enjoyed teaching, though the conditions were exploitative and the salary abysmal, and found the students engaged and serious. I felt that I had a mission in life.

My pregnancy was healthy and my weight gain good. I experienced no morning sickness and went back to a vegan diet. Early in the pregnancy, I began having the most amazingly numinous and prophetic dreams. In these dreams I was visited by little Black girls; sometimes they were babies, other times, toddlers. In one dream, a little girl, about three years old, came and held my hands. Her face looked like one of my sisters, but I knew I did not know her. I asked her who she was and she promptly announced, "I am your daughter." In yet another dream I came home from work and found a baby, about five months old, lying on my bed. We conversed, and again she told me that I was her mother. But the language we spoke was an ancient Ethiopian tongue. Thus, right from the beginning of the pregnancy, I knew I carried a female child. In all these dreams the baby was surrounded by and bathed in a beautiful light. I would later give as a middle name Noor to the child in my womb. Noor means "sacred light" in Arabic. In the Qur'an there is a surah called An-Noor, the words of which I tell my daughter are her power words.

February was the birth month of this child. February was also the middle month of the second term, so I knew I had to get my course covered while I was away on the very short maternity leave that the university gave to teaching assistants. The students gave me cards and a few also gave me gifts for the baby.

I got my classes covered, and on the evening of Friday, February 12, I left the Robarts Library, where I was doing research. I went to the bank at the corner of Bay and Bloor and did a transaction. All the while I was wrapped in the knowledge that the child in me was beginning the journey of its descent. After twelve years my body had forgotten a lot and felt new, almost as if it were my first birth. Contractions rippled across my belly. I drove home, one hand on the wheel and the other on my belly, rubbing it.

When I got home, I told my husband to ready the house. I think it is a fanatical Jamaican thing, having the house clean and tidy in preparation for a birth. I called my sister Charmaine (she had emigrated two years before) and told her that the baby would come soon. I also called my midwife and alerted her that labour would be beginning.

Yes, the midwife. The Bob Rae NDP government was in power and had passed legislation empowering midwives and home births. Anyone wishing such a birth and service, however, had to pay from one's own pocket. Though I could have given birth in a hospital with the midwives in attendance, I opted for a home birth.

The reason I did not have a hospital birth this time around was simple. The obstetrician that my family doctor referred me to worked at a famous downtown hospital. During the few visits I had with her I did not like her. Her manner was brusque, and she dealt with me as if I were an object. I was also told that the hospital kept the mother and child for not more than forty-eight hours. Hospitals needed beds, and why keep a woman and her child around when both were okay? Many women and their babies leave the day after the birth, the nurse who was giving the tour told me. She also said it was what many of the new mothers preferred.

I thought to myself, why leave my home for a few hours, give birth, and then hustle back home? I would rather have the child in the comfort of my home, where I could do as I pleased.

Anne, my midwife, was wise and knowledgeable, and she loved her job. I trusted her implicitly. Anne had told me what to get for the home birth: disposable bedsheets and pads, eight pillows, hot water bottles, white grape juice, glucose, Bach Rescue Remedy (to take the mother out of shock), and a host of other supplies.

All day Saturday I had "baby pains." By 1:00 a.m. Sunday morning, my water had broken and the labour began in earnest. Something happened too that had not happened with my first birth — I vomited over and over. The midwives arrived at 3:30 a.m. and Anne ran a warm bath. She submerged me in the water where I laboured for most of the time. Beneath the water the contractions were gentle. Whenever I raised my body into the dry air, the contractions were intense and painful. I did not want to leave the bath. I sang and cried. I moaned and groaned. I recited poetry from memory.

Around 7:00 a.m. Anne took me from the bath. On the bed, waves and waves of pain washed over me. I focused on my breath. I had never concentrated on anything so intensely in my life. Again, focusing on the breath carried me through labour.

Two friends, Gabriella and Debbie, arrived with a video camera. In between contractions I told them to set it up and to shoot the scenes. I had the midwives giving testimony, and my husband, Alpha; Akil, who was now eleven and a half; and, of course, I spoke to the camera. Looking back on that event, I think I must have been nuts: there I was directing a video shoot in the middle of my labour!

I was tiring. The midwife gave me Rescue Remedy, and I drank grape juice to keep up my energy. My friends talked about this and that to distract me. Alpha followed the midwives' instructions to boil various things in water. Finally, Anne got me up from the bed and whipped out her birthing stool. She instructed me to squat over the stool. She said I had laboured long enough. It appeared that the labour was stalled. Lying on my back on the bed was helping none—I needed the assistance of gravity. Squatting over the birthing stool would ensure that my body would naturally push the baby down while gravity would likewise exert its pull. So I squatted, as millions of women have done for millennia. I thought of Atabeyra, mother goddess of the Caribbean Tainos, and the petroglyphs of her in caves in St. Vincent and other Caribbean countries as she squats and pushes a child from her loins. Gravity worked. The baby's head crowned. Anne said it looked like a big head, and it appeared to be stuck. Anne massaged my perineum. I contrast this action to the one twelve years before, when the young doctor was ready to cut me open with a knife. Anne massaged the area gently and was the first to see the head emerge.

"The head is coming!" she shouted excitedly.

A contraction washed over me. I pushed big. I moaned, but still managed to ask the videographer if she was getting the shot.

"The shoulders are coming out!"

By this time I was having an out-of-body experience. I felt my spirit leaving my body. I could still push and speak, cry and moan, but I felt my spirit leaving my body. I observed all that was going on, was very present and completely aware, but seemed removed from the experience. Time seemed to have stopped.

The baby slid out, and we all cried and laughed at the same time. An eleven-hour marathon! I was sore and bleeding. Anne held up the child and gave it to me. It was a girl. I put her wet and naked body on top of mine. Our breathing synchronized.

She was perfection. Her eyes were black pools of water. She was alert, and light came from her face. Anne waited a while before she had the umbilical cord cut, and Alpha did the honours. She was eight pounds, twelve ounces. A big baby. No wonder her head got stuck in the birth canal!

Because we are Muslims, her father took her aside and whispered the azan in her ears. The azan is the call to prayer. It is done at the moment of birth, in hopes that the child will lead a prayerful life in connection to the Creator. I also wiped honey on her lips. Honey, the first taste she would experience in her life, and a symbol that her days would be more sweet than bitter.

I looked at my new baby. A mass of curly hair covered her head. She had a round forehead and chubby cheeks. She looked like a cherub. Pretty and sweet. I put her to the breast and she sucked greedily.

It was February 14, Valentine's Day. I could not have asked for a better Valentine's Day present.

BY THE TIME I GAVE birth to my third child and second daughter, Habiba, I was thirty-eight years old and had put on a lot of weight from a sedentary lifestyle. I was attempting to write a doctoral dissertation while teaching at the same time. At the end of my pregnancy with her I weighed 172 pounds. The doctor and midwives assured me this was normal for my height of five feet, six inches. But if I worried about my weight, it was from vanity, because my health was perfect. I exercised and enjoyed swimming. I swam right into my ninth month.

I got pregnant with Habiba at a time during my menstrual cycle when I was not supposed to get pregnant. But, as I would discover with this child, she had a mind and mission of her own. When my period did not come, I did not bother to go to the doctor for a test; I knew I was pregnant, because my period was as regular as clockwork.

The pregnancy came at a time when I was at a crossroads in my life. The marriage had become difficult, and I had entertained thoughts of dissolving it. I was stuck in my doctoral studies, which was becoming financially untenable. I was always broke. The support and mentoring I needed for my work was not forthcoming from my professors. I felt I was on my own, trying to do the impossible.

The sexism in the academic system was clear. At least two of my male colleagues had pregnant wives, but no one commented on that. It was assumed that they would carry their studies to a conclusion without being interrupted by "female problems." The graduate departments of academe were still constructed as male spaces in which women were intruders. The people in my department pretended not to see my growing belly. I did not receive one word of encouragement or support.

Because of my school and marriage issues, I knew that this pregnancy was going to be a journey of faith and love. I also knew that things happen for a reason. Everything in its time and place. This pregnancy came at an "awkward" time, but really the timing was perfect. It was meant to be. I felt it in my bones. And more than anything else, I wanted this baby.

Without thinking about it, or even being very aware of it, I was playing the role of superwoman, or the strong Black woman. I was teaching, researching, planning a dissertation, and married with two young children, with another on the way. And I was doing all of this with very limited financial resources. My scholarship money had run out. The pay for a teaching assistant was next to nothing.

My husband's earnings as a small business owner were not

enough to see us through. If I allowed myself to think about the problems, I would get depressed. But I visualized the light and beauty at the end of the journey, and I prayed and meditated. I drew on the energies of my ancestors.

And I was making history. I would be the first Black woman at the University of Toronto to complete a graduate degree in Canadian history.

During this pregnancy I also entered a heightened state of spiritual awareness. My dreams were numinous. In several dreams I was visited by the presence of Mary, the mother of Jesus (I gave my daughter the middle name Mariam in honour of these dreams). I learnt new surahs. My prayers were steadfast. I took various seminars on healing and meditation. It was during one such seminar that the name for the child came to me.

It was towards the end of March, and I was attending a "tools for healing" workshop at the Swansea Town Hall in Toronto. The workshop leader was a woman from Scottsdale, Arizona. She was teaching things like muscle testing, harmonic overtones, dowsing, and so on. She took us through a meditation exercise, and at the end of it, sitting in peaceful repose, I heard the name whispered to me. "Her name is Habiba." The voice was as clear as the song of a bird. It repeated the message: "Her name is Habiba." I smiled to myself. *Habiba* is Arabic for "beloved." And what a fitting name. Because the decision to have this child, and loving her and my pregnancy, and doing my best to ensure a safe and empowering delivery were indeed acts of love.

I also prepared for the birth in other crucial ways. I remembered when Lamarana first began nursing, how sensitive my nipples were and how they felt when her lips clamped down on them. So I prepared my nipples for such an eventuality with Habiba.

In Jamaica, in the last few months of a woman's pregnancy, she would leave her breasts bare. It is believed that the dry air will help harden the nipples. She would also use a hair comb on the nipples, so that when the baby began sucking, they would not be soft and sensitive. Having hard nipples was an asset. If a woman's nipples were too soft, they would become sore and blistered from constant sucking.

I too aired and combed my nipples when I was about seven months pregnant. I also prepared myself for an easy birth by eating copious amounts of okra. Jamaican women believe that if a pregnant woman eats lots of okra, the slimy juice from the plant will help the baby slide out of the birth canal with little or no pain to the mother or child. I also drank a particular herbal tea that was supposed to relax the muscles of the birth canal and make birthing easy.

Habiba's labour began at the university. I often tell people that both my daughters were born in the library. During my pregnancies I read, researched, taught, argued, and discussed with students and professors, and so I believe some of that intellectual acuity and awareness went into the genes of the children. I went home and prepared myself. My partner was out of the country on a family emergency. His best friend, Yasin, came over, sat with me, and was a great support. I rubbed my belly and focused on my breath as tiny contractions rippled across my belly. At 1:00 a.m. on Saturday, April 6, 1996, I decided to go to bed and get some sleep. I could not sleep, and by 1:30 the contractions were coming every five minutes. I waited until they were coming at three minute intervals before I woke up Yasin and told him to call the midwives. They lived close by and were there by 2:00 a.m. I called my sister Charmaine, and she came in a cab with her daughter Shelley. There was no video camera this time, but Shelley was armed with a 35-millimetre camera. I had three loving and capable midwives, and my sister Charmaine was a nurse. I was in good hands. Akil and Lamarana were asleep. I decided not to wake them.

Katrina, the head midwife, ran a warm bath and submerged me in it. The contractions were forceful and intense. One thing was different about Habiba's labour. There was really no pre-labour and very little time between contractions, which came one right after the other. Katrina said the birth would be fast.

Finally, at 5:00 a.m. Katrina took me from the bath and to the bed. As I walked to the bed, a strong contraction ripped through my body. The midwife felt it and held me.

"I love you," I said to her. And I meant it. I felt love coursing through my entire being. It was a light and heady feeling. I felt love for everyone in the room. I felt love pouring from every part of me into every part of the child who was on her journey to be born. The feeling of love was overwhelming.

When I lay on the bed, my water broke. It was greenish and full of mucus. It gushed onto my legs and over the bed. I was in an elemental space. And the out-of-body experience that I had felt at the birth of Lamarana came back, but this time in full force. I observed everyone, my senses were keen, yet it felt like I was flying above it all. I surrendered myself to the pain. I entered through the gateway of pain and became one with it, and in doing so, I conquered it.

"Push." It was Katrina's voice. She massaged my perineum. "The baby is coming," she said.

My sister held my hands. Sweat poured from my body. I looked through the narrow window and saw dawn coming in the eastern sky. Pink and orange clouds emerging from dark ones.

"Push."

I turned my head to look at the blue bottle I had used for several months as a focal point for breathing. Blue, I was told and had read, was a colour that calmed the mind and regularized the breath. I looked at the bottle and breathed and pushed, and suddenly everything went black. The lights had gone out. And in that instant the bottle fell from the shelf and smashed. The lights came back on and the baby slid out of my vagina. I looked at the clock. It was 5:30 a.m.

The entire labour lasted for four and a half hours. It was my shortest and most intense labour. Slipping from my womb, Habiba was still partially covered in her protective sac, what Jamaicans call the caul. It seemed that she emerged from the caul only at the hour of her birth. *Hmm,* I thought to myself. In Afro-Jamaican tradition a child born with a caul is felt to have special powers. The midwives cleaned her off and weighed her — seven pounds, eight ounces. A good size. The baby latched on to the nipple, and the milk came right away.

"What a way to announce yourself to the world!" Elizabeth, the assistant midwife, said. "She is a warrior."

I looked at the nursing baby: her facial structure was already outlined, her forehead and cheekbones prominent. Her eyelashes were long and dark, and she had that famous pouty upper lip from her mother's side. Even if she was going to be a Boadicea, Aisha bint Abu Bakr, Anacaona, Queen Nzingha, Nanny, or Harriet Tubman, she was also going to be a great beauty.

WHAT THEY NEGLECT TO MENTION

Claire Wilkshire

SOME WOMEN ENJOY BEING PREGNANT. Good for them. I remember rage — betrayal! All the things they never warned you about. It was a cabal. If they told you the truth, no one would have babies. So they lied a bit, they omitted much. Once you were waddling around with a hand clamped to your lower back, bumping into the furniture that kept coming closer, then you started finding out about all the little details no one saw fit to mention until it was far too late. A friend said, "I wouldn't say I had pain exactly. Discomfort, yes, but not really pain." I believed her.

It's like ocean view or not. "Not" means soup cans piled up in a back alley. In the birth tourist literature, labour is all ocean views. But when you get to the delivery room, the soup cans start heaving into view.

It was a sunny Friday afternoon at Grace Hospital in St. John's. I could talk only to Larry. People would say things like, Hi, this is X and this is Y . . . in the nursing program . . . opportunity to observe . . . The talking would go on for a while, then Larry would look at me and say, She's having a contraction now, just wait a minute. And in a bit he would say, What do you think, and I would make one kind of moanish grunt and he'd say, She doesn't mind but just one of you if that's okay, which is exactly what the grunt was meant to convey. How he managed this I have never been sure.

I knelt on the tile floor with my face pressed against the metal bar of the bed, thinking, *I didn't know it would hurt this much, I don't think I can cope, I have changed my mind, I have been misinformed, I would like a complaint form, I can't go through with it.* It was, of course, too late then. That was the scariest part, knowing the worst was on the way and wondering how bad it was going to be.

I did not choose the path of virtuous suffering. Suffering terrified me. I wanted drugs and I said so. They gave me one lot, but by the time it wore off, the labour was more advanced, the contractions earth-shattering. Then they said, Well, you can't actually have any more because it's a funny thing about the drug: it doesn't work more than once. If you have a second shot, it makes the pain worse. What bastard, I wondered — sock-footed and yellow-gowned and all twisty-faced — invented a drug that would work for a brief period, and then, when you needed it even more urgently, would suddenly have the opposite effect? Why did they not see fit to mention this before Dose One? Was this the best they could do?

It was.

Except that, of course, as agreed, you could have an epidural. If you feel it is too much pain, all you have to do is say you want an epidural — they've made this clear — and it's yours.

I want an epidural, I said clearly. It is too much pain.

It will slow down your labour, that's the only thing, they said, so it will take longer.

I don't care, I want the epidural. How soon can—

Well, actually, you are going to have the baby in not too long, and by the time the anesthetist got set up, you'd already be having the baby, so there's not much point.

I think it will feel like too long to me, and I want the epidural anyway; you said I could.

The thing is, the anesthetist isn't available right at the moment, and when she comes you'll probably —

Are you saying I can't have an epidural?

Yes.

And there are no more drugs.

Right.

I hate you all.

(I never said that about the hating. They were all nice, they were wonderful; they just didn't seem to realize how much deception was going on.)

What else don't they tell you? Oh, if you do not own a hair dryer then you should pop out and get one. Guess why. For your stitches. But not on High, they say with a smile; it's their little joke, haha, bloody sadists. Did I mention they were all very nice?

Other little secrets you discover: afterpains. That's when you basically go through labour all over again, but this time the baby is already born and your family has gone home and the doctors are in bed and it's just you and the night nurse, and she has a bunch of other people to take care of. But not to worry: it's good news! It means your uterus is expelling the goop and going back to normal size, so you should just lie back and rejoice in the sensation of disembowelment.

After my son was born I had a shower, which they seemed to consider bizarre, risk-taking behaviour; they insisted on wheeling me down the hall. I swished all the slimy stuff off with huge relief, and a nervous voice just around the tiled corner kept saying, Are you all right in there?

Phyllis came at night to visit and brought a cold beer. I made the mistake of asking if I could drink it and discovered that I wasn't allowed because of the painkillers for the afterpains, but I kept it hidden in a cool spot on the window ledge, behind the curtain, something only I knew about. It was a kind of talisman.

And then of course there are hemorrhoids: they seem slightly funny until you've had them. I saw a young mother position a rubber tire on her chair and ease herself down onto it very, very carefully. By then I already knew it wasn't funny.

It's not all about labour, though. You forget most of that stuff. Larry says he can't remember any of it, although that's probably not true. One thing it's about is transformation. You are transformed from a person into a person who is a parent.

My first Mother's Day was a few weeks after the birth of my son. Mothers, I thought contemptuously. (No offence to any mothers; it's just that I'd pretty much maxed out on the whole idea by then.) And a moment later I realized that was what I was: a mother. It came as a complete surprise. I was becoming another sort of person.

You need to become the sort of person who can do the things that you need to do.

Last year my son climbed on a cannon by the waterfront on the French island of St. Pierre, off the south coast of Newfoundland. My daughter climbed on the other one and jumped off into my arms. She clambered back up and jumped again as my son looked on. I walked over to his cannon and spread my arms out.

Go ahead, I said.

My son was eleven. He eyed me and then the ground.

Nah, he said.

I can catch you, I said. I was thinking: I think I can catch him—I can try. If he jumps, I will have to catch him, and that's all there is to it.

I don't really feel like it, he said, sounding resigned.

Come *on*, I said, and he hesitated and then jumped. I caught him and squeezed him tight and deposited him on the ground, and he was grinning. Will you catch me again?

The thing about birth is that it's not really about birth, it's not about labour and delivery. It's about what happens after. It's about the fact that seven years later a girl tears across the playground when she sees me coming. Pink and red flowers on her white capris, T-shirt and sun hat and sturdy, filthy sneakers: she's going full tilt, so fast she skids through the gravel, a huge grin revealing the hole where one front tooth was until last week, and because of the skid she slams into me hard and I almost topple over backwards. She wraps her arms around my waist and squeezes, tips her face up and beams and says: Mumma!! The curious fact that this small, grubby person with two long braids—a man at the Wal-Mart checkout once reached out and grasped them in one hand because he just couldn't stop himself, because he had granddaughters—the fact that this person adores me and that my arrival gives her great pleasure and that the feeling is mutual... that's what birth must be about, surely.

NEW EYES, NEW HEART

Karen Connelly

ALWAYS THE STRUGGLE OF the living is to be born.

Birth is the first crisis—in the Greek sense of the word, meaning "point of decision," not disaster, as we often think of it—the crucial turning point in existence, the great turning out of the amniotic sea, that inner ocean that rocks and sways in red darkness, red light.

Before birth, there is no separation. There is only joining. First the divided flesh, two human bodies naked and hungry and hopefully willing, hopefully razzle-dazzle. We think of lovemaking as the culmination of human passion, but the most fervent, ambitious, and headlong passion happens beyond our reckoning. The sperm rushes in and the egg responds to that lucky wriggling by enveloping it whole. Genetic ecstasy begins in a little sea around the zygote. While we are brushing our teeth. Or falling asleep.

Thousands of new cells divide only to join further. Within a month, the fine net of the nervous system is already sprouted, the brain a future bud *ectoderm endoderm mesoderm*, the gastrointestinal tract is making itself up like perfect jazz *da-bi-bab-BOOM*, the

blood and muscles are waving flags *go go go*, and it all goes, shocking machine, marvellously, quickly; the pancreas and liver snap
into cellular relief, and here is an imagining of bones, as angular
and soft as the word *skel e tuuuun*. In just a few weeks more, the
pumping heart is moored under ribs as fine as a hummingbird's.
The deep muscles of the psoas and the iliacus stretch from the
lower vertebrae all the way down to the lesser trochanters of
two tiny inner thighs.

The pregnant woman is an earth unto herself, and her season is relentless spring. She may be joyful with it, or furious, or
depressed, or proud. Most likely she is all of these and more.

I STOPPED ON THE ROAD to regard the valley tumbling down to
the sea in all its rich July fertility — apricots ripened and fallen,
olives hard nubs on the silver-backed trees, watermelons plump
and naked under the sun. I put one hand on my belly. Seven
months. The blue Aegean shimmered against the paler blue sky.
I announced to the olive groves: I am building his eyes so he will
see this valley.

Then, more humbly, hedging my bets — I was in Greece,
after all, where hubris has a history, and who really knew
what child I was growing? Maybe he would be blind — I said,
like an old Greek woman, God willing. Then, like an ancient
Greek woman, Goddess willing. I invoked Artemis, the Lady
of Creatures. Her torso is covered in breasts so she can nourish the world; animals walk on her shoulders and nestle at her
waist and in the crooks of her arms. Yet such is the measure
of her greatness that she is also the goddess of the hunt, an
unrepentant taker of life. Both creator and destroyer, she is an
embodiment of every human mother's power. Her Ephesian
temple was so extraordinary that it was considered one of the

seven wonders of the ancient world, when Ephesus was still on the edge of the sea.

Thump and *swish* went the little fish; Minnow we called him, our own sea creature. A knee or a foot bumped the inner wall of my aquarium. The creature inside me flipped entire. Whenever he somersaulted like that—I called him "he" though I didn't know the sex—I thought of how much work it was going to be to push him out. Again came that phrase, the little mantra that had coursed through my mind since the beginning of my pregnancy: *always the struggle of the living is to be born.* The baby was so strong in the womb that even though he was part of me, I knew he was also himself. I was in awe of him.

It was happy awe. This was the golden age: months five, six, and seven. My husband was far away in Canada, so it was just us, myself and Minnow. I swam every day in the Aegean, two or three times, and in the little beachfront tavernas I ate grilled sardines and lamb. The villagers were full of admiration, as they tend to be for pregnant women—the fertility cult of Artemis lives on even now—and at least a dozen old men and women predicted from the shape of my belly that the child was a boy.

Though my lower back was killing me, I often walked the mile down to the village. I sang a song for Artemis on the high open point of the dirt road. Then, because the beauty of the valley encourages prayer, I stood still and whispered, O Artemis, mother of the world, hear my prayer (women two thousand years ago said this; every willingly pregnant woman on the planet wishes this): Please keep the baby safe. Please protect pregnant women in all their vulnerability. Please protect me. Help my body be strong for the coming birth. Help this baby come easily and quickly and safely into the world.

It is possible that Artemis was not listening. More likely she has, like most deities, a mysterious sense of humour.

And when it comes to birth, there is only so much a goddess can do. If the struggle of the living is to be born, then the pregnant woman's struggle is to be born anew with the baby she is bearing, as the mother of a new child; to be born as one who no longer controls. And birth is just the beginning.

I WAS AT HOME IN Toronto when I went into labour. After my husband, Robert, and I had timed the contractions to make sure they were coming regularly enough—and on they came, mildly but steadily, through the night—Robert called the midwife in the morning.

She was not the midwife who had attended me throughout my pregnancy. My midwife was away, at a conference in Ottawa. I had predicted I would go into labour the weekend she was away, and so I did. I was trying to be philosophical about this change, but I was disappointed.

The whole point of having a midwife was to develop a more personal relationship with the caregiver who would guide us through a home birth. Home, in our own bed—or on the floor, if I felt like it—seemed like the right place for me to have a healthy baby. My mother had laboured all five of her babies at home as long as she could, then rushed to the hospital when she knew she was close. If she had been slightly older, or younger and a hippy, she would have had home births too—except for my older brother, who was breech. But even the breech birth she did on her own, without drugs or painkillers. My mother disliked the hospital because "someone is always interrupting you," and she maintained that you needed a little peace and a lot of elbow grease to have a baby. She was my inspiration.

Robert continued talking to the midwife. He was nodding too much. He covered the phone with his palm. "She says you need to make sure this isn't false labour. She's suggesting that you take a bath." A hot bath will often send prelabour contractions ebbing away.

My irritation flared into anger. The strength of my response was confounding, though I didn't think of that at the time. I wanted so badly to be in labour, and though the suggestion that I take a bath was perfectly reasonable, it felt to me like an expression of disbelief. Did she think I was *lying*?

In my most petulant, childish voice, I snapped, "What if I don't *want* to take a bath?"

He conveyed this question, minus the angry pout, to the midwife, and came back with an alternative. "She says you could take a hot shower instead. Just to make sure."

Make sure of what? That I was telling the trúth? This was *my* body, after all; I knew what was happening. Why wouldn't they believe me?

We walked slowly up the stairs, Robert behind me, shepherding me, supporting me — which is what he did through the following hours, generously, beautifully. We went into the bathroom. He gently asked, "So ... do you want to take a bath or a shower?"

"Bath!"

I could barely speak, partly because of the contractions, but also ... also because ... I didn't know why. The clenching in my lower belly had settled slightly, which made me think that the midwife's call had interrupted the rhythm of the contractions. But still they came on, those deep, raking waves, the low pain that made me go still and quiet. I sat on the toilet to pee. Robert turned on the bathtub taps and went into the other room.

Suddenly, without knowing what was happening, I started to scream, "I don't want to take a bath, I don't want to take a bath!" I was still sitting in the alcove on the toilet, pressing my hands against the walls as another contraction came over me, uncontrollable and steady and not really so hard, but this time it was localized as a stabbing pain in my vagina. In the middle of such an intense contraction I couldn't stand up, I couldn't escape. The walls on either side were pressing against me; I was being suffocated, crushed.

I was screaming loudly now, without words, in the full grip not of early labour pains but of a very unexpected episode of traumatic re-enactment. It had been years since I'd had such a strong flashback — encompassing, transforming, turning my adult woman's body into the body of a child again, a toddler's body, a baby's; without language. And in pure terror of the bath-tub. That was the site where, for some years, I was abused.

When a flashback comes so suddenly, it is like going insane in the space of a minute. If a person did not know what was happening to her, she would think, *Yes, I've come to the end of my mind; I've just lost it*, when, curiously enough, the opposite is true. The mind is finally arriving in the body, finding out, unburying the truth in the flesh.

I had worked with a therapist; I knew I was not crazy. But I was hypersensitive from sleep deprivation and the hormonal surges of early labour. I quickly realized why all that stuff about *not being believed* by the midwife had upset me so much. For many years I had struggled to believe consciously what my body had always known.

As I apprehended what was taking place, the sensations began to dissipate — much like a contraction releasing, letting go its hard grip on the deep muscle. But I was crying now, and trying not to hyperventilate. And I was overwhelmed by a powerful desire to get the hell out of the bathroom.

The bathroom in our house has two doors. One opens into the master bedroom and the other one opens into my office. I managed to turn off the bathtub taps before I stumbled out.

My husband found me on our bed, covering one eye, then the other—a form of trauma therapy that uses the eyes to work with the left and right sides of the brain. Some day, I thought, I will write about this remarkable form of physical therapy; some day I will write explicitly about sexual abuse and the work of heal-ing trauma, not only in a personal context but also in the global one, because I have come to believe that we live in increasingly traumatized societies, small and large human families locked in ancient cycles of violence and denial, damaging not only each other but the planet we live on.

But now I had to gather my strength and focus again, return fully to my body. I gently reminded myself, *You are not the baby.*

Seeing that my breath had steadied, Robert asked, "Can you take a bath?"

I was calmer now, though every few minutes a contraction held me still and drew a deep groan out of me. The baby stuck his elbow out, kicked downward; I felt the new weight of his head pushing hard on my bladder. Whether it took one hour or twelve, our little fish was swimming away, pushing his way out. "I'll get in the tub. Can you bring me a glass of water?"

Robert helped me lower myself into the warm water. It eased the pain of the contractions without stopping them. Once out of the tub, I walked around the top floor of the house. The waves through my uterus got stronger. I kept walking, around and around, out of the bedroom, past the stairway and wooden rail-ing into the office, through the bathroom, back into the bedroom.

I groaned loudly as the contractions intensified, often leaning over on the writing desk in the office, where I had done so much groaning in the past. My back labour was intense too, more difficult to bear sometimes than the contractions, but Robert greatly alleviated that pain by pressing against my lower back.

The midwives, Katrina and Nicole, arrived and checked my cervix. Katrina was the presiding midwife; Nicole was a student, almost finished her training. They were both surprised: I was already dilated six centimetres. *See?* I thought. *I told you I was in labour.* They checked the fetal heart rate. The only thing that wasn't quite up to speed was my water: it hadn't broken yet. But the baby and I were coping well with the work of labour. The midwives went downstairs to the kitchen to have some lunch and wait. I preferred to labour on my own, with Robert bringing me food and various drinks. It was an intense, quiet, and very intimate time for us. We took a shower together; we talked. We laboured together sometimes, and sometimes I just wanted to be alone.

Later in the afternoon the midwives came back up to assess us again — everything normal — then checked my cervix. Katrina wanted to try to feel the baby's skull, to see what position he was in. It is fiercely uncomfortable to have a stranger put most of her hand in your vagina, then stick a finger into your cervix. She wasn't absolutely sure of what she felt, because my water still hadn't broken.

"I want you to consider letting me break your water," she said, and explained that she would do this by inserting a small hook into the cervix and pricking the amniotic sac. In the past couple of hours I hadn't dilated much more; she impressed upon me that labour wasn't progressing as quickly as it ought to. Rupturing the amniotic sac would get the contractions going more quickly.

"Let's wait a couple more hours," I said. I was highly suspicious of any fiddling. It felt wrong. The water would break when it was time. So far, everything had been fine. Though I was tired, having not slept the night before, I felt I could handle quite a few more hours of contractions.

LATE AFTERNOON, I LOOKED OUT the window at the tall tree, in the full yellow regalia of autumn, as vivid as the forsythia had been months before. I was waiting intently for the next contraction, but before it came, I said to Robert, "Imagine if we experienced our whole lives with such attention, paying homage to every moment. What would it be to live that way?"

Robert, being himself, made a joke. I can't remember what he said, but I laughed. A little while later Katrina told me that she didn't think my contractions were strong enough. If you can laugh between them, apparently, you're not in hard labour.

It felt pretty hard to me. During those waves my body felt like it was rearing up, wrenching up from the belly outward; the centre was opening slowly. I had been doing a lot of squatting, simply because it felt good and alleviated some of the intense pain in my back. Katrina suggested that I try some side-lying to intensify and regularize the rhythm of the contractions.

Now that was pain. I was prone, on my right. The contractions immediately became longer and stronger, bigger, the way waves come up huge and hurl you down, leave you wrung out with a mouth full of sand, stunned. My groans grew into deep, low roars, belly in the throat — my belly was my whole body. A baby was in there, held tight, pressing down as the cervix spread, opened into my uterus, and the uterus became, or wanted to become, part of the birth canal, pushing the baby out, moment by moment, into the world. The pain was immense but manageable, focused. It was what I had expected. There was time to breathe and rest between contractions. It was not the frightening pain of sudden injury but the pain of work: the good, hard pain of labour. My mind was loosened and concentrated at the same time, pure animal. The whole time, I was impressed by what my strong body was going through. But it was taking so long.

I let Katrina rupture the amniotic sac at six o'clock. It didn't hurt at all, and there wasn't as much water as I expected. It also didn't have much effect. I thought the contractions were going to become immensely more painful and intense still, but they didn't.

It began to get dark; then it was dark. I had been in labour for twenty-four hours, still without any sleep. The last time Katrina checked my cervix, I had not dilated past seven centimetres. She checked me again, struggled again to feel the baby's fontanels, those little gaps in the plates of skull that seem to be sutured together. The fontanel at the front of the head is diamond-shaped; at the back, it's triangular. Katrina believed that the baby hadn't turned the right way. A caput had formed on that recalcitrant little head—a swelling from the pressure against the cervix. She also felt that my cervix was slightly closed because of the atypical pressure of the baby's head.

Then I heard those words you never learn in prenatal class. Transverse. Asynclitic. Posterior. Instead of lying face down towards my spine, ready to tuck his chin down and slide out like a reasonable baby, he was lying face-up, as if looking through my belly at the ceiling, and his head was turned towards my thigh. In this position the baby was presenting the greatest diameter of his head to my cervix.

I thought, with a grumpy dose of irony, *Always the struggle of the living to be born.* No kidding. For the first time Katrina mentioned the word *hospital*.

MANY, MANY MONTHS LATER — this month, in fact, now that my child is ten months old and walking, with a head that still turns, unexpectedly and stubbornly, in all sorts of directions — I look up all these words on the Internet and read about how to turn an asynclitic, transverse-arrested, or posterior baby. I learn that rupturing the amniotic sac can be the worst thing to do, as it can commit the baby more fully to the atypical position and make turning him more difficult. I learn that the polar-bear position for labour — knees to chest, ass up in the air — can often get the baby to turn. And doing lunges and pancakes — switching back and forth into and out of a variety of birth positions — also can work very well. I read that side-lying on the left — not the right — can sometimes "spin a baby."

But on October 18, 2006, I was in deep but unproductive labour, and not about to sit at my computer and look up some alternatives to what the midwife was suggesting. After all, she had been catching babies for fifteen years. She made it clear that she thought we should go to the hospital. Secondarily, with little enthusiasm or conviction, she suggested the possibility of doing nipple stimulation to release more oxytocin — which might increase my contractions — or doing lunges, which might help the baby rotate. But she felt that the best thing to do was make a trip down the street, to Mount Sinai Hospital. She also said that if I had an epidural, I might get a chance to sleep.

Around this time I had a great urge to push, but I could not push because I wasn't fully dilated. Minnow couldn't get out. I didn't know what else to do. With a great heavy heart and an aggravating sense of failure — *Should I just stay put, wait more, change positions? I should never have let her break my water* — I started getting ready for the hospital.

We already had a small bag packed, just in case, but I needed a couple of other things. A favourite black stone. My little white sculpture, Cycladic, of a pregnant woman holding her ancient belly. I didn't want to go to the hospital without a single talisman, a respectful nod to the goddess.

THE MIDWIFE'S IDEA OF having a rest at the hospital was like a cruel joke. Just getting strapped into the fetal monitor was a nightmare, and having to lie down to accommodate the strap made the contractions more uncomfortable.

Nicole tried to put the IV in my hand, but she could not find a big enough vein. Every time the needle went in it brought on another contraction. The needle seemed to be scraping bone. After a couple of tries, I asked her to call a nurse to do it. But the nurse had a hard time too. At one point she proclaimed, "You're a pregnant woman; your veins are supposed to be swollen." Finally she managed to insert the needle. I needed the IV for the Pitocin drip, and because that medication makes contractions gut-wrenchingly powerful, Katrina also recommended that I have an epidural. This suggestion upset me. I knew that an epidural greatly increases a woman's likelihood of more intervention, often leading, for various reasons, to a Caesarean birth.

Deferring to the midwife's experience, I decided to go ahead. But going ahead in the busy maternity ward of a large Canadian hospital late at night is not so simple. The anesthesiologist who was to administer the epidural was busy. Until he was ready to do the epidural, we couldn't get the Pitocin going. In the meantime I started running a low-grade fever, which is not uncommon when labour has been interrupted and the woman is getting dehydrated. I had eaten and drunk all through my hours at home, but in the hospital, women in labour are still denied these privileges in case they end up having to go into surgery. Robert gave me water on the sly; the midwives turned their heads. Though I was receiving fluids through the IV, I still felt thirsty.

For the first time I began to get discouraged. My contractions started to weaken. There were just too many interruptions and discomforts. I remember thinking how amazing it was that most women *want* to go to the hospital to have their babies; it was the last place I wanted to be. When the anesthesiologist finally arrived, I grilled him about what the epidural would do to me, to the baby, to the labour. The answers were thorough; he even began anticipating the questions. Then a nurse came in and said to him, "That woman who's just had the C-section is screaming her head off—she's in agony."

He looked at me apologetically. I said, "Clearly she needs you more than I do." So he went away again for a while. Then he came back and had me sign the release form, which basically said that I wouldn't hold the hospital responsible if something went wrong with the epidural, which can cause paralysis if not administered properly. I signed. He had me sit up straight to insert the needle and, like Nicole and the nurse with my hands, he couldn't find the right vein. He inserted the needle a couple of times and dug around between my lower vertebrae, all the while telling me—as I had an unexpectedly strong contraction, brought on again by the pain of the needle insertion—to sit very still, because otherwise he risked damaging a nerve in my back.

The needle was eventually inserted, and the effect of the drug was almost immediate. The contractions continued but I couldn't feel them very much now. Then the Pitocin drip was administered to strengthen the contractions.

After the first flush of Pitocin, the baby's heart began to decelerate. Katrina went off to consult with the obstetrician on the floor, Dr. Thomas. I talked to Robert about how awful

I was feeling. And furious. I knew heart decelerations were serious; I was scared for the baby. Was it the Pitocin that caused the
deceleration, or the epidural? Who knew? It didn't really matter.
Minnow had been ready to come out, trying to come out, for
many hours now. What was happening to him in there?

Katrina came back with a grim, tired face. She turned off the
Pitocin, because the contractions were proving too much for
the baby to handle. For the first time she talked to me about a
Caesarean section. "I think it's important that you know what it
will be like. They'll drape your body with surgical sheets. Your
arms will be laid straight out, away from your sides. The incision
is here" — she showed me on her lower belly — "and it's about
this long, into the uterus. Then they take the baby out…"

Finally, I cried. This was everything I did not want. The hospital and its culture, all these interventions, the drugs. I wanted
to feel my own pain. And the waiting and struggling and fiddling
was to end only in the ultimate unnatural birth: surgery. I was so
sad. And exhausted. And there was absolutely nothing I could do.
I could not stop the birth and begin all over again. Poor Minnow
was stuck and he simply had to come out, soon.

I looked at my mysterious Cycladic woman, perfectly serene
and pregnant and marble — she was sitting on top of the grey
metal locker where our coats were hanging — and I cried quietly,
because I didn't have the strength to howl.

The midwife checked the fetal monitor again. With my weeping, the baby's heart rate had bounced back to normal. I was still
crying, but we all started to laugh as well. Katrina left the room
again to consult with the doctor.

A few minutes later, the obstetrician arrived. She was an
attractive, down-to-earth brunette in her mid-forties. She was
a proverbial breath of fresh air. While the rest of us were worn

out from attending this long labour, Dr. Thomas sailed in, raised her open hands in the air as if to say, Who knows why it's such a struggle? and announced, "Listen, this guy's gotta come out soon, even if it's a C-section. You need to hold this baby in the next hour." She made the possibility of the surgery seem less depressing. She was full of energy but also calm, matter-of-fact. I knew that if she laughed she would have a big, contagious laugh. She quickly took a blood sample from the baby's scalp—which was right there, dammit, so close and yet so far—to check the carbon monoxide content, to make sure he still had enough oxygen. He did; she gave the okay for the Pitocin to be turned on again.

Half an hour later Katrina took a look inside me. I watched her face between my spread knees: her eyebrows went up. She was genuinely surprised, and sounded confused. "I can't believe this, but you're fully dilated. The baby must have turned. I'll just ask Dr. Thomas if she wants to insert a fetal scalp monitor, to make sure he's still all right."

She ran off and returned with Dr. Thomas, who took a quick look between my legs and hooted. Then I heard the big, generous laugh that I knew she would have. "Fetal scalp monitor? Ha! This baby is coming out *now!*"

The doctor then looked up at me and smiled hugely. She could have left then, but she stayed. She stood by me and held her hands on my enormous belly, feeling my contractions for me. Robert stood on my other side, holding my hand.

The moment she said, "Push!" everyone else in the room— my husband, Katrina, and Nicole—joined in as her chorus and yelled, "Push, push!" I pushed, all through myself, outward. My weariness had disappeared. I was thrilled to be able to use my strength. Finally!

The doctor said to Katrina, "Look at that: she knows how to

push! Even with the epidural!" She smiled at me again. "It's like you've had a baby before! It's great, you know exactly what to do. Now, now, again, push!" Up went the rallying cry from everyone once more: "Push!"

"Put your hands between your legs to feel the head crowning."

I put my hands there and announced, with enormous pleasure, "He's like a wet kitten, there's so much hair."

Nicole said, "Okay, now pant, little pants, little pushes." This was to keep my perineum from tearing too much. "Slowly, slowly. Now get ready for another big push."

I closed my eyes to push as hard as I could. But Dr. Thomas said, "Open your eyes and watch your baby get born." Out he came, little Timo Jo Sup Connelly Chang—all seven pounds and nine ounces of him—in a great tide of blood and amniotic fluid. He didn't cry immediately; they took him to the warmer and gave him a scrub to get him going. Then up went that shocking new voice in our lives, that siren of aliveness and need. A minute later, one of the midwives placed him on my chest. He was indeed a boy, fulfilling the predictions of my Greek villagers. Little squalling boy body, all arms and legs wriggling against me. He cried, he screamed; it was gorgeous. Within a few minutes he was suckling my left breast—still his favourite.

A sense of pure exultation filled the room, filled each one of us. Katrina and Nicole were so happy, and deeply relieved; I was laughing every few minutes; Robert and I kept smiling and touching each other. This sense of achievement kept us all going for the next two hours until, just after seven in the morning, Robert and I brought Timo home, where we had wanted to be all along. My elation—that I had pushed my son out on my own, that I had avoided a Caesarean—lasted for several hours more, then faded as exhaustion took over. We slept; we ate; we marvelled at Timo, who was black-haired and dark-eyed already, and beautiful, and strange, and fiercely hungry. And not much of a sleeper.

The next day I discussed the monumental change of birth plans with *my* midwife, who had returned from her conference. What could have been done differently? Was I at fault somehow? Should I have laboured longer at home? Done some jumping jacks? These were inevitable and necessary questions, asked in the midst of the sweet, mind-numbing delight and chaos of Timo's arrival. Over the next couple of weeks, watching him and learning how to take care of him, I created a new story for the birth that was and let go of my regret for the birth that wasn't.

Always the struggle of the living is to be born. And the birth of new eyes and a new heart is always a triumph.

DRIVING LESSONS

Joseph Boyden

NEW ORLEANS, 2004

The heat of the day has given way to an inky, balmy Louisiana night, our car windows rolled down as we speed, tires humming on pavement, along Bienville Street. Amanda accelerates through the yellow light at Carollton, me bitching. "See," I say, almost gloating as she brakes hard on the quiet, dark road for a man in the middle of it in front of us. "You keep speeding and cops'll get us."

The man in the street, black against the black asphalt and wearing a white T-shirt, looks up, looks into our headlights. He's struggling, right there in our lane, with something at his feet. Dropped groceries. A sack of something large. Not another car or person in sight, just Amanda and me and this man ahead. We stop in front of him. He's not a man at all but a teen, his eyes wide open, caught in some embarrassing act, staring into our lights. It's not dropped groceries he's struggling with, we see, but another young man sitting down in the road.

We are close enough to see blood on the sitter's blue shirt. The young one on top drags his charge out of our way to the

111

curb. Amanda pulls up beside the two, and I'm going to ask them if they're all right, if they need some help. The kid on the ground must be drunk. He's fallen on the road, head lolling, and his friend is helping him get out of our way, keeping him safe from the white, too-fast drivers.

What happens next happens in seconds. But to this day it plays out in my head like a lifetime. My arm hangs out the window, close enough to reach and touch them. I am about to open my mouth when I see that the standing teen has a pistol in his hand. He looks at me, eyes cold now, and begins to raise the gun towards us. I shout to Amanda, "He's got a gun! Drivedrivedrive!" In the very instant she peels away, I see the kid change his mind, lower the gun. He points it at the head of the one below him and pulls the trigger. I watch the barrel flash, hear the gun pop. Doesn't sound loud at all. He turns then and runs, fast as he can, down a side street.

Not half a block away, I scream, "Stopstopstop!" Amanda doesn't want to. I scream again. She does. "I saw which way he went," I shout, opening the door and bolting. "No!" Amanda panics. I go, running, then stopping, worried about the return of the shooter. I barely hear Amanda yelling into the row of dark houses, "Call 911! Call 911!" I stare down the side street, look to see if the shooter will come back. Will kill me. I run to the man on the ground. He looks so small. He lies on his side, in fetal position, eyes staring at the dirty blacktop. He panics when I approach. He whines like a baby with a stomach ache, begins to hyperventilate when I kneel.

"I'm not him," I whisper. "It's okay."

I stroke his hair and he calms. His whine becomes a moan. He stares out at the road, waiting. I sit down and put his head on my lap. I stroke his head like he's my child. "It's okay. You're going to be okay." I hum to cover his moan, to relax him. He's bleeding out, I see, his blue shirt soaked black in the streetlight, blood running out of him and puddling by the curb. He's shot in the chest. I consider mouth-to-mouth, but only for a second. He's dying, and there's nothing anyone can do about it. Only then do I see the bullet hole, neat and round, in his cheek. I stroke his head and whisper, "You're okay. You're going to be okay. Just breathe." I think he takes some solace in my words. The panic has turned to resolve. To calm. I hum some more, continue stroking his head. His short black hair is wiry, greasy. He's as thin as my son, who will be fourteen next month. But this one on the ground, bleeding on me, he's clearly a few years older. His breathing slows. "You're going to be okay. Just breathe," I whisper, I hum, as his eyes glass over and he dies in my lap.

—◠

TORONTO, 1990

We're stuck in rush-hour traffic at 8:30 a.m. on Sheppard Avenue in North York. She turned nineteen last month. I am twenty-three, won't meet Amanda for another two years.

We are in the back seat of a Buick Skylark. She's sprawled on the seat, naked. I crouch awkwardly between her spread legs. She's screaming. Her mother, who's driving, screams as well. I look up for a moment, out the window, and see the shocked expression of a woman staring back at me from another car.

Our car inches forwards, horn blaring, and I look back down. Blood. Lots of it, on the seat. *That will never come out*, I think. *Upholstery is ruined*. White noise in my head like a TV that's set to a blank station at full volume. I'm sure this girl is dying. She screams more. A blood-smeared round lump pushes out from her body. The head of my child. She yelps, and the lump pushes out further.

My eyes watch all of this unfold, my brain numb with horror. But my hands, they are calm and steady. The hands of my long-dead surgeon father. The blood-smeared mass spits out fast from her body, and my hands catch it and stop it from slipping onto the floor.

The little thing is long and skinny, It's blue in the harsh morning light. The umbilical cord is wrapped tightly about its neck. It doesn't move, doesn't cry, doesn't breathe. I see all of this, am shocked to blankness to see all of this. But the hands, they work steadily, unwinding the umbilical cord. The body is slippery. *Don't drop it.*

Now it begins to gasp a little, but something still prevents it from drawing breath. The pointer finger of my left hand prods the tiny mouth open, scoops out bile and goo. The hands turn the baby onto its stomach. While the right hand cradles it, the left hand gives a quick slap to the tiny rump. The baby gasps, begins to draw in more breath, bleats like a lamb. The bleats turn into wails. The blue skin begins to turn pink.

I watch as one hand gently wipes some blood from the child. The other hand makes a nest of the mother's robe on her puffed stomach. Both hands lay the baby gently in the robe to keep it warm. The baby screams full-fledged now, its lungs clear and obviously strong. Its mother lies back with eyes closed, breathing easier, passed out. The new grandmother honks her way through traffic and speeds to the Emergency Room entrance of North York General. I haven't even noticed if my child is a boy or a girl.

We settle, two days later, on the name Jacob. Despite the protests of family on both sides, I decide that his middle name will be Buick. I like to drive him through the dark streets of my neighbourhood at night. He is loud, healthy, and only calms each evening to the hum of car tires on pavement.

EARTH MOTHER

Joan Clark

HYPNOTIZED AND SIX MONTHS pregnant, I am sitting in the obstetrician's office with my eyes closed, my back against the outer office door. The doctor is saying, "You are very, very relaxed and thinking about the birth of your baby. It will be an easy birth, and you will be as relaxed as you are now." I am relaxed, sublimely, weightlessly relaxed, listening to the doctor's persuasive voice while simultaneously listening to the receptionist on the other side of the door. In a heightened state of being, I hear every word she says to admitting patients, as well as every word the doctor says. He's about to count backwards from ten, and when he reaches one, I will no longer be hypnotized. Though incapable of lifting my pinkie from the arm of the chair without his instruction, I say, "But it's lovely sitting here. Let me stay." I am unwilling to leave this state of perfect bliss. "You can't stay. You have to go. I have other patients to see," he says, and begins to count.

A WARM JULY AFTERNOON. My sister and brother-in-law are visiting from Toronto and we are having tea in the backyard of our tiny rented house. Seven months pregnant, I am sitting on the grass, bare arms looped around my legs, cradling my belly. Morning sickness is far behind and I am blooming with health, with the voluptuous ripeness of my body. The baby kicks, and around us bees suck up the nectar of honeysuckle and mock orange. I am in an erotic trance; without a word to our guests, I drift into the house and peel off my clothes. My husband follows and we make love in the bedroom off the kitchen, the sheer blue curtain billowing like a sail, sweeping the sweet, seductive scent of honeysuckle and mock orange across our nakedness. The voices of my sister and her husband blur with the hum of bees on the other side of the screen.

———

IT IS 1966. Nine and a half months pregnant, I am lying on the surgical bed of the operating room. On the other side of the bed are metal stirrups to hold my heels when the time comes, and higher up on the bed, metal wings where my wrists will be strapped down. A light as big as a flying saucer's beams down. At the edge of my vision are stainless steel instruments and unspecified tools. I'm lying on my side, knees up. I'm seized by a gargantuan contraction; a moan rises from my gut and I gasp with the effort of riding out the pain. My in-a-hurry son can't break out of the womb fast enough. I have an urge to push hard to help him out, but the nurse locks my knees together and warns me not to. "The doctor's on his way," she says. "It won't be long now." Desperate to push, I ask if she can help me deliver the baby. "Afraid not," she says, patting my knees. "Doctor's orders."

I AM IN ANOTHER OBSTETRICIAN'S office, in a strange city, two months after my first son, an encephalic, died at birth. I am here for a checkup and reassurance. I tell the doctor that I was advised not to get pregnant again for at least six months. "Though with the odds being what they are," I say, "it's unlikely that I will have another encephalic."

The doctor peers at me through horn-rimmed glasses. "On the contrary, you are more likely than most women to have another freak."

Dressed for the occasion, I am wearing a turquoise cotton dress with white polka dots and white low-heeled shoes. As I clutch my handbag, my knees shake uncontrollably and I focus on the office door, trying to figure out if I am capable of wrenching it open and getting out of there fast.

I AM IN THE MEDIEVAL labour room of Holy Cross Hospital in Calgary. Four other women and one girl are in the room, each of us lying on a utilitarian metal bed, a crucifix on the wall above, white hospital curtains separating us. I am on the bed next to the window. The woman on the bed one over from mine groans whenever a contraction grabs her. In the bed opposite her, a woman, seized by a wave of pain, curses her husband. "You fucker!" she yells. "You got me into this!" The other two women are quiet. Perhaps, like me, they are listening.

Across from me a priest sits on a metal chair, taking confession from an eighteen-year-old girl. She has already confessed that the father of her baby is the father of the children she was hired to look after. She sobs, gulps back tears. She has a breech birth ahead of her, yet the priest continues to sit and prod. What does he want? Does he want her to confess the sin of being seduced?

———

IT IS THE FIRST of four trips to the Holy Cross Hospital to give birth to my moonstruck son. In the labour room my doctor pulls the white curtain around us so that the two of us occupy an intimate space. Sitting on the bed, he begins to hypnotize me. "Breathe deeply and relax," he says. "Whenever you feel a contraction, breathe deeply and relax." Over and over he repeats this mantra and willingly I obey. As long as I am relaxed, the contraction is nothing more than a massive stretching, as if a wide elastic band were being pulled across my belly. The doctor begins to count, pulling me deeper and deeper into a trance. When he reaches one, he lifts first my arm and then my leg, letting them flop onto the bed. "You are completely relaxed," he says and triumphant, goes off to find a hospital bed on which he can nap until summoned by a nurse.

———

MY MOTHER WAS A nurse. She gave birth to me at home, upstairs on the marital bed, my sister asleep in the next room, my father making lawn furniture in the basement. Because the doctor was on an out-of-town call, my mother asked a friend, also a nurse, to help. Like my sister's birth, mine took only a few hours. My slender mother, the doctor was fond of saying, was like a racehorse.

I was two weeks overdue, and to wake me up to the fact that it was time to be born, my mother instructed Ila, her nurse friend, to drive us over the notoriously rugged Western Head Road, to be sure not to miss a rut or a pothole. After the drive my mother went down the basement stairs and jumped off the fourth step, trying to jolt me out of my dreaming, to awaken me to the fact that I could not linger in her womb forever. I was born a few hours later, my mother said, pink and white.

———

LIKE ME, MY CHILDREN love hearing stories of their births: how their father and I, on the fourth trip to the hospital, walked around it—one large city block—for hours before the contractions petered out and, disconsolate, we returned home. How moments after his birth, my blue-eyed son opened his eyes and peed on my belly. How black my son's eyes were at birth, his hands roundly fisted, his ears plastered to his dark, wet head. How, after a phone call that announced our daughter had arrived, we drove through every red light on Twelfth Avenue to reach her.

———

MY DAUGHTER IS ADOPTED, and for me her birth was opening the door of a fourth-floor office and seeing our three-month-old, grey-eyed daughter, chubby knees drawn up as she lay on a pink blanket spread on the social worker's desk. Our daughter smiled as if she had been waiting for us all along. When I picked her up and carried her to the car, she snuggled into the hollow beneath my neck, as if she understood she was going home to the room where elephants and monkeys frolicked on the walls in a pale wash of pastel colours.

———

BEFORE MY ENCEPHALIC SON was wrenched from the birth canal, a sheet was draped over my knees to prevent me from viewing the deformed head. No sheet was required for the two subsequent births. Both times my healthy sons, only seconds old, their heads slick with slime, were placed on my belly, I said, "Isn't he beautiful?" I am awed by the miracle of their being. The wonder of the baby, kicking and shifting himself inside my belly these past months, now here, on the outside of me. A baby with a well-shaped head, ten fingers, ten toes. Perfect in every way. Proud of us both and anesthetized by rapture, I don't even feel the doctor stitching me up. Pain is no longer a word I recognize — discomfort, yes, but not pain.

———

IN THE DOCTOR'S OFFICE six weeks after the birth of my moonstruck son, I wondered aloud about the mysterious duality of pain, how quickly its iron fist unclenches after birth. The obstetrician-hypnotist grinned. "That's because you were hypnotized," he said. Because I had become fond of the obstetrician-hypnotist (later to become a psychiatrist), I let it go. But I am still amazed that he could persuade himself that I was hypnotized during the birth of my blue-eyed son, who was born after my legs were held together while I waited for the man now sitting opposite me to show up. Was this his way of laying claim to an experience he would never have himself?

———

If I had to choose a word that for me would encapsulate birth, it would be *joy*. Joy, joyous, joyful. No single word can describe the glorious feeling that attends a successful birth, whether it be a child born from my body or from another woman's. After our black-eyed son was born, I refused to sleep and for three days floated close to the ceiling in hormonal ecstasy. High on the ether of giving birth to a healthy baby boy, I resisted diluting even a particle of joy. Meanwhile my husband was explaining that the blister on his lip was the result of having put the lit end of a cigarette in his mouth after he heard the joyful news — during the 1960s fathers were not admitted to birthing rooms and were told the news by a doctor or nurse.

IN THE MONTHS BEFORE giving birth, I had, like so many pregnant women, gone through the preparatory rituals of fixing up the baby's room, painting furniture and papering walls, filling drawers with sleepers and vests, stacks of diapers. I read Dr. Spock, whose book in 1966 was a mother's bible. I was wholly focused on the baby and was taken completely by surprise when birth transformed me into a mother bear, a creature of instinct, watchful, fierce, ever on the alert for real and imagined threats and dangers. The ferocity of maternal love took me by surprise. It was visceral, primeval. Although my children are grown, the instinct to nourish and protect, to hold them within my paws, is with me still.

MY SONS COULD HAVE been conceived inside a tent or on a beach but as it happened, they were conceived on the marital bed in a room that later became another kind of labour room: the room where I wrote. There are many ways of giving birth, and following the birth of my black-eyed son, I gave birth to what amazingly became my first book. I wrote on a desk in the corner of our bedroom, and continued to do so during my children's growing-up years. Though I now have the luxury of writing in a room of my own, part of me misses using my office bedroom at a time in my life when mothering and writing fiction were one.

—

DRIVING PAST ST. CLARE'S Hospital, I see a hugely pregnant woman on the sidewalk, supported by her baby's father. I watch as they turn off LeMarchant Street onto Campbell Avenue. Like a pregnant Cree woman following the travois, or me walking around the Holy Cross Hospital, my husband's hand supporting my elbow, the woman is preoccupied, her concentration on the strenuous stretch of muscle across her own belly. She looks frightened, but resolute and determined. Inside the car, the seatbelt stretched across my own belly, I visualize the cataclysmic, earthquakian power of her body and imagine her opening up, spreading herself wide, emptying herself of water and blood as she delivers a miraculous new being to the earth.

NOT A NATURAL CHILDBIRTH STORY

Edeet Ravel

SATURDAY, JUNE 20

I am thirty-two today. I am also basically two people. I love being two people. How much closer can you get to someone than having them right inside you? Also, I love this other person. I have loved her madly for exactly thirty-six weeks. And soon, very soon, I'll get to meet her.

Meanwhile, I'm calling to confirm with the movers. When your due date is July 3, it is not a good idea to move house on July 1, but this is Montreal, and July 1 is moving day. If you're due to give birth two days after you move, that's just your bad luck.

SUNDAY, JUNE 21

I do not—repeat, *do not*—believe in astrology. Unless, of course, there is a scientific basis to astral influences that we haven't discovered yet. Until then, I am a non-believer.

Nevertheless, wouldn't it be nice if Larissa were born when the moon was in Libra? Such a lovely place for the moon to be. I mean, even if there's nothing to it—and there *isn't*, as far as

we know (which maybe isn't very far)—it can't hurt to be born
when the moon is well placed, can it?

I wouldn't have known when the moon was going to
be in Libra, or what that could possibly mean, but John, my
CP-member, math-genius, Lukács-expert husband, told me. How
he came to know anything about astrology is one of those mys-
teries that must remain forever unsolved. In fact, he pointed out
that if conception took place on October 3, everything would be
favourably aligned thirty-eight weeks later. So October 3 it was.

It's worked out exactly as planned. Larissa will no doubt be
born exactly on my due date, July 3, because the moon goes into
Libra at nine or ten that morning. Twelve days to go!

MONDAY, JUNE 22
There's no going back! There's only one way for Larissa to come
out! It's not a good way! Nature goofed! And now I'm stuck.
Help!

Okay, time to reread *Spiritual Midwifery*. Childbirth is a won-
drous, spiritual experience. It's going to be great. Really great.
Really, really great. Yes, it is.

TUESDAY, JUNE 23
John and I have not chosen a boy's name. I never did have the
second ultrasound, so I don't in fact know whether I'm going
to have a girl, but John and I are certain nonetheless. When you
want a girl this much, it's not possible to have a boy.

One of the reasons I want a girl is the circumcision problem. I can't even think about the circumcision problem. John
wasn't circumcised (in case the Nazis came again). So now not
being circumcised is still weird, but maybe not *that* weird, while
circumcision is still not really barbaric, but maybe it's a *little*

barbaric—either way, the idea of my poor little baby in distress is entirely unbearable. Luckily I won't have to deal with any of this, because I'm going to have a girl.

Another reason is that, given the way our marriage is faring, I don't think we'll have another child. The past nine months have not been promising, to say the least. And if I'm to have only one child (I was hoping for five, but the best-laid plans, etc.), I would really, really like to have a daughter. You always know what to give a daughter on her birthday, and you can brush her hair at night.

Nine days to go.

THURSDAY, JUNE 25
My parents have left for Israel and won't be back until July 5, which means they won't be around when the moon goes into Libra. This is what happens when you give birth to the second grandchild.

John's parents, on the other hand, are hoping to pick up my daughter a few minutes after she's born and look after her, at their place, for the next several years.

FRIDAY, JUNE 26
I am staring at the photographs in *Spiritual Midwifery* when it suddenly occurs to me that even though I am planning to have natural childbirth, *I don't have a coach!*

John has only one phobia and, just my luck, it's related to pain. He inherited the condition from his father, who developed it following his three-year incarceration in one of Stalin's prisons.

If John so much as hears about pain, he has to leave the room so as not to pass out. This pretty much rules him out as coach. I phone Mrs. Allie, my prenatal class teacher, who's also a midwife, and she says she'll be happy to help me out. She tells me to phone her when I enter the second part of labour. Labour, like pregnancy, apparently has three parts.

I'm happy, I think. I like Mrs. Allie — though I don't really know her. She seems nice, and she knows all about massage and so on, and she loves midwifery — but what if she doesn't feel sufficiently sorry for me?

No, no, Mrs. Allie is perfect. I've learned her breathing techniques, she'll know how dilated I am, she's totally reliable, and she isn't militant. I don't want anyone militant, just in case.

SATURDAY, JUNE 27
Why, why didn't I explore the hypnosis option?

SUNDAY, JUNE 28
Larissa's heel is pushing against my stomach. I can see its shape very clearly. Is that cute or what? Oh, I can't wait to kiss that little heel!

MONDAY, JUNE 29
Or the acupuncture option . . .

WEDNESDAY, JULY 1
John and four guys from Kahnawake move all our things from a one-bedroom apartment with no washing-machine outlet (on Drolet) to a two-bedroom apartment with a washing-machine outlet (on Berri).

I watch them from the sidewalk like a great moored ship surrounded by sailors on shore leave.

When the movers depart, John and I realize we can't possibly get sufficiently organized to spend the night in the new place.

We move into my parents' empty apartment for the night.

Thursday, July 2

2:00 p.m.

I'm on my doctor's examining table for a checkup. My doctor is the incomparable Dr. Eason. Erica Eason is without doubt the nicest, smartest, most committed obstetrician in Montreal, and probably the world, and she's one of only two or three in Canada who insist on attending the births of their patients.

She listens to my stomach. "Hmm, you're in labour," she informs me.

Well, that's good news. I thought labour hurt, and clearly it doesn't. This is going to be a breeze.

Dr. Eason tells me to go home and relax.

5:00 p.m.

I don't believe it: I've come down with a cold. It's the cold John's had all week, which I was sure I wouldn't catch from him because whoever heard of going into labour with a cold? How are you supposed to do breathing exercises with a stuffed nose?

Never mind. Even with a cold I'm going to have a joyous, electrifying, spiritual experience.

9:00 p.m.

I've watched *Cheers* and *Family Ties* on my parents' TV. We don't own a TV so I've never seen either show before. I didn't know sitcoms could be so captivating.

While absorbed in popular culture, I consume an entire container of tofu ice cream.

John is at the new place, trying desperately to set up the bed.

11:00 p.m.

John shows up. I tell him I'm having vague contractions. He tries to convince me to go to the hospital.

"There's lots of time," I assure him.

John has visions of having to deliver the baby in the back seat of our little blue Colt.

"Don't worry," I tell him. "It'll be hours before I give birth." The books were right: labour can be fun. I go to sleep.

FRIDAY, JULY 3

1:00 a.m.

My stuffed-up nose wakes me up.

Okay, I guess we can go to the hospital now, even though the contractions are quite far apart and I can still barely feel them. But we may as well get the trip over with.

I take the little bag of things I'll need, along with Mrs. Allie's phone number. We start out in the little blue Colt, John still convinced I'm going to give birth while he's driving down Decarie Boulevard. After one block I ask him to turn back. I want more tofu ice cream.

"You're kidding," John says hopefully.

"I'm having a craving." We head back, I eat a bowl of ice cream, and we set out again.

2:00 a.m.

I'm wearing a hospital gown and trying to produce a urine sample in a small toilet at the Royal Victoria Hospital. As I try to aim into the little container without getting my thighs and feet wet, a new sensation—commonly known, I think, as pain—takes me by surprise. What the—?

Okay, don't panic. Remember *Spiritual Midwifery*. Remember

all those prenatal class movies. This is an exciting, positive experience. I'm going to take a walk with John. That white hospital gown they've given him is very becoming. He should have been a doctor, I've always said so.

2:15 a.m.
John and I are walking up and down the hall. Everything's under control.

2:17 a.m.
"Get me a chair!!" I scream.

2:30 a.m.
I am very, very lucky. They've given me the birthing room, seeing as I'm going to have a natural childbirth. It's a very nice room. John asks me whether I want to listen to the tape I've brought with me, Janet Baker singing Mahler. I look at him and wonder if he's insane.

2:40 a.m.
I am informed that I'm in the first stage of labour. I am not interested.

2:42 a.m.
My water hasn't broken. An intern comes to attend to the matter. The procedure is entirely painless, as far as I can tell.

2:55 a.m.
I am hooked up to a machine that tells me when I'm having a contraction. Good thing I have that.

3:40 a.m.

John shakes his head.

"You actually thought you'd be listening to music," he says incredulously.

So far he has not fainted. He's even taken my hand. However, I have no one to breathe with. If only we could call Mrs. Allie, but it's the middle of the night and I'm still in the first stage of labour, apparently.

3:50 a.m.

The best explanation for the way I feel now is that it's the sixteenth century and someone who thinks I'm a witch is trying to extract a confession.

On the other hand, between contractions I feel great.

4:10 a.m.

Lord, Lord, let there be drugs.

4:20 a.m.

How come my pain is all in my back? Has something gone horribly wrong? John is instructed to find a nurse and seek an answer.

4:30 a.m.

"Back labour," a nurse says knowingly. "That's what I had too. Felt it all in my back."

I guess that's reassuring.

4:35 a.m.

It has come to the nurses' attention that I am not being coached. They are amazed. They had assumed, when I said I was doing natural childbirth and had taken the course, and when they saw that my husband was with me, that said husband was my coach.

Now it seems I have no coach, I am not breathing with any-one, and my husband is sitting beside me like a bump on a log.

The situation might have come to the nurses' attention ear-lier, but I haven't made a sound. This is not because I'm stoic; it's because I have a sensitive throat, and screaming hurts my vocal cords. However, it would be interesting to see my face during contractions. What's that movie, with the guy travelling through time and what it does to his mouth? Too bad we don't have a video camera.

4:45 a.m.
A coaching nurse is sent in to help me.

4:50 a.m.
This breathing is good! Why wasn't I breathing up until now? This breathing is fantastic. It really helps. I hardly felt this contraction. The breathing nurse is great! I love her! Breathe in, blow out, look into her eyes. I love her, I love her! I'll do anything for her, anything she ever asks of me. Oh, nurse, don't leave me. *Don't ever leave me.*

5:15 a.m.
The coaching nurse leaves me. It's the end of her shift.

5:35 a.m.
The members of the St Martin in the Fields Chorus come to find out, one by one, what a cervix at this stage of labour feels like.

John, if not an ideal coach, is at least a good person to have by your side while the tenor section—I mean students—checks your cervix. When the cervix inspectors first enter the room, he rises from his chair and looks at the door with longing. He even turns towards the door, but then decides to stand by me instead and stroke my arm lovingly.

Yes, John is stroking my arm lovingly! Send in the entire hospital to check my cervix! Bring them on!

Oh God, I'm going to have a child with a man who has never stroked my arm or any other part of me lovingly until now. I may have made a small error...

6:10 a.m.
John falls asleep in his chair.

6:40 a.m.
John lets out a blood-curdling cry in his sleep. He is no doubt dreaming that he is in a room with a hundred women in labour, all expecting him to do something about it.

7:00 a.m.
Epidural, epidural, epidural. The most beautiful word in the English language. *"Do not call Mrs. Allie. Did you call her?"* I inquire with some urgency.

"No," John replies calmly.

"Don't call her!" I repeat, relieved. "Tell them I want the epidural."

John goes to deliver the message. We are both under the mistaken impression that I can have the epidural immediately and therefore don't need Mrs. Allie to get me through the next God-knows-how-many hours until I'm ready for it.

All that reading, and I don't even know the basics! And alas, there is no one to enlighten me.

7:20 a.m.

John returns with a nurse.

"We called Dr. Eason," the nurse says. "She says you want natural childbirth."

These words bring on the worst contraction yet.

"It's some great misunderstanding," I assure her when it's over.

7:40 a.m.

The nurse returns to tell me that Dr. Eason is on her way.

"Does she live far?" I whine piteously, still under the mistaken notion that getting the epidural depends on Dr. Eason's arrival.

For some reason I suddenly remember my father warning me about that whine. "No one will marry you if you whine like that," he said. "They'll just hear that whine and turn away."

"No, no, she's just across the street," the nurse replies.

"Oh, can't you get another doctor to agree?" I whine even more piteously.

"She'll be here very soon," the nurse says, still not aware of the misapprehension under which I am literally labouring—that Dr. Eason, not dilation, is all that lies between me and drugs.

7:50 a.m.

John looks depressed. However, he has not yet passed out, so that's good.

8:07 a.m.

Dr. Eason is hovering over me.

"She's pretty uncomfortable," the first nurse says. Uncomfortable! I have to remember that one next time I teach my class the meaning of the word *euphemism*.

"I hear you're asking for an epidural," she says.

"Yes," I say meekly.

"You're sure you're not just feeling isolated?" she asks.

I am feeling isolated, now that she's mentioned it. I'm feeling both pain and isolation, and, may I add, isolation because of pain. Because of pain and because of *no one to breathe with me.*

"Yes, I'm sure," I say.

"Well, you're not dilated enough yet. You have to be four centimetres dilated, and you're only at two."

This would be a good time to call Mrs. Allie, but we don't, maybe because I'm vaguely worried that Mrs. Allie will try to talk me out of having an epidural, but more probably because John and I just aren't thinking.

"We can give you Demerol," Dr. Eason offers.

Demerol! A street drug! An epidural is bad enough, but Demerol *reaches the fetus.* I'm not going to inflict a *street drug* on my innocent baby!

"Does Demerol reach the baby?" I ask in a tiny voice, hoping that between yesterday and this morning there have been essential modifications to the laws of physics.

"Yes, the baby goes to sleep immediately," she says.

"Okay, I'll have some," I say.

8:40 a.m.

Do not take Demerol during labour.

First, you will immediately puke up all the tofu ice cream you ate earlier. You will puke into the container provided for that purpose and then you will puke all over the floor.

Then you will get very sleepy. You'll feel your contractions, but now you'll be sleepy on top of that.

Not relaxed, just sleepy.

Only you won't be able to go to sleep. You'll be in too much pain.

Instead, *make sure someone is there to breathe with you!*

11:10 a.m.

A very delicate blonde intern, with very delicate, thin fingers (please keep this plot element in mind), arrives to check my cervix.

"Say four, say four," I whisper in a manic mantra. "Say four," I repeat more loudly.

The intern says, "Yes, you're four centimetres dilated now."

There is a God.

11:25 a.m.

John goes to inform the powers that be that I am ready for my epidural. He returns with three people: a nurse, a very cheerful anesthetist with an Australian (or South African) accent, and a student.

A student! A student is going to give me the epidural, and it's obviously his first time! If it goes wrong I will be paralyzed for life. I could even die. And this student is huge; he looks like a sumo wrestler, and he has very, very stubby fingers. Why me, why me?

"Ready?" the anesthetist asks with incredible optimism and good humour.

"Yes," I say, obediently sitting up and bending forward.

"Good. Very good," the cheerful anesthetist tells the student as he runs his (stubby) fingers along my back.

"Good, good," I repeat inanely. Everything is good. It is good that he is doing a good job, it is good that the cheerful anesthetist is being so encouraging, it is especially good that soon I will feel no pain.

11:30 a.m.
I didn't feel a thing. And the sumo wrestler apparently got it right.

11:40 a.m.
No pain. I am drifting off.

5:30 p.m.
I have slept for six hours. Poor John has been to our new place to wait for the washing machine, which was due to arrive in the afternoon. Where are friends and family when you need them?

A doctor with a moustache and large hands comes to check my cervix again.

"Four? Who said four? You're barely two centimetres dilated."

5:40 p.m.
Dr. Eason reappears. She's not at all pleased with the staff. How could they not make absolutely certain I was ready before giving me the epidural?

What she doesn't know is that it was my fault. I broke the delicate blonde intern with my pitiful whining.

"You'll have to be induced now," the nurse informs me.

5:55 p.m.
I am attached to a fetal heart monitor on one side, an IV on the other. A large machine measures the drug going into the IV, which is going through my shoulder to my back, or something.

9:00 p.m.
I am in a bad mood. This entire labour has been a fiasco! I refuse to push. I'm sulking. Nothing else has gone right, why should this be the exception?

"Push," Dr. Eason is saying. I blow up my cheeks, squeeze my eyes shut, and pretend to push. My silence gives me away.

"Groan!" Dr. Eason tells me.

I groan, but I'm still faking.

Besides, how can I push if I can't feel anything? Besides, if I push I might get hemorrhoids. Why take a chance?

Also I am dying, I mean dying of thirst. Every few seconds I yell, "Ice! " and John hands me a cup of crushed ice.

How thirsty can a human being possibly be?

The nurses don't think I should drink. But Dr. Eason says, "Let her have a glass of water." Instead of sipping slowly, I gulp it all at once and promptly puke again.

11:00 p.m.

Erica Eason has given up on me. I'm not pushing, I'm in a bad mood, I'm whining again—and this is the real thing, this is masterful, accomplished whining—and, thanks to an acidic stomach, my breath could fell an army. In the entire history of the Royal Victoria Hospital, no one has experienced anything like it. Only John can't smell my breath. He still has that cold, and his nose is blocked.

"We'll try forceps, but we'll prepare for a Caesarean," Dr. Eason decides.

Good, I'm glad. Let's just get this over with.

11:14 p.m.

Dr. Eason assures John, who's thinking of eighteenth-century novels, that the forceps go on the baby's shoulder. Then she calls in another doctor for a second opinion.

"Isn't it awful what women go through?" he says kindly.

"Isn't it great how strong women are?" Dr. Eason, my hero forever, replies.

The cheerful anesthetist comes in again and gives me a new drug. Now I'll be frozen from the waist down.

"Will it harm the baby?" I ask, to ensure my popularity.

"Of course not," she says, laughing. "That's why we're not living in the jungle, dear." Everyone loves the cheerful anesthetist from South Africa (or Australia), and I can see why. But I'm still nervous. They used to think a lot of things were okay that turned out not to be okay. And what does that mean—*that's why we're not living in the jungle*—so that we can pretend we know everything?

I look in the mirror above me and see Dr. Eason's hand going in for one last try without forceps. *So that's why she has such long, beautiful hands*, I think in a slightly stoned way. I shut my eyes and decide to push. Yes, I'm going to push, finally.

11:19 p.m.
Everyone exclaims. "Good push! It's a girl!"

I open my eyes. After all that, I missed seeing Larissa coming out.

"Lovely, healthy cry," Dr. Eason says proudly.

I try to look at Larissa but I can't lift my head. I also can't feel her on my belly. She's been taken away for cleaning and eye drops.

11:25 p.m.
I glance again at the mirror and see the placenta coming out. Interesting, if you enjoy seeing what could be the grey brain of an alien coming out of you, but actually I could have done without that bit.

I turn to John. I have never, in my entire life, seen anyone look so relieved.

Where is my baby, for God's sake?

11:27 p.m.

Larissa is finally handed to me. Oh, oh, oh, oh, oh, bliss! Oh, bliss and more bliss! I love her! I love her I love her I love her!

I cover Larissa and myself with the blanket. She immediately opens her eyes and looks left and right, wondering where she is. Brilliant!

"Hi, Larissa," I say, and I can tell she's heard me.

11:35 p.m.

I hand Larissa to John. He's nervous about holding her, but he takes her, and his eyes fill with love for this little baby of his.

I'll never be unhappy again, ever. I may not manage to make things work with this complicated guy, I may have all sorts of misfortunes, but no matter my how imperfect my life is, Larissa, who *is* perfect, will fill my heart with gladness.

THE BABY LISTENS

Anne Fleming

THE DUE DATE — December 6 — comes and goes. Okay, the baby will not have the day of the Montreal massacre for a birthday. Fine. Good. Phew.

December 7 comes and goes.

December 8.

December 9.

December 10.

We could not be off in our calculations. We know exactly when this baby was conceived: March 9, 11:00 a.m. That's when the nurse wrangled the syringe full of Donor 3139's sperm past a tricky cervix right into the uterus to meet Cindy's newly dropped egg (whose monthly arrival Cindy had been graphing for the past half-year via mucus phases, spikes in daily basal temperature, and faint-striped ovulation kits).

March 9.

One month later I came home from Ontario, where my mother had just been admitted to hospital with pneumonia and a strange dementia in which she seemed to have a dual consciousness. One consciousness madly plucked non-existent buttons off the table; the other knew the buttons didn't exist but couldn't stop the first. There was a good chance she was dying. Cindy met me at the airport. "I think I'm pregnant," she said. All I could think about was my dying mother, my distraught father, neither of whom had any idea we were trying to have a child. Who, I was guessing, would not be receptive to this pregnancy. Okay, would be actively antipathetic towards this pregnancy. Whose antipathy towards this pregnancy was one factor in the ten-year delay between our first talking about having a kid and deciding to actually do it. My mom might come around, but she was seeing goblins pop out from behind cars. She was in no state to take in the information. My dad? Oy.

Home from the airport, Cindy took the test. Yup, pregnant.

After the first trimester I told my parents.

"Steer a long way from thinking of us as grandparents," my father said.

"Speak for yourself," said my mom.

DECEMBER 11 COMES AND goes. The baby is five days overdue. Nothing to worry about. Nothing unusual. Cindy is finished work. I'm finished teaching for the term. Nothing to do but mark portfolios and wait. Our friends Mary and Jackie are doing the same thing in Toronto, waiting for their baby to be born.

Six months earlier we hadn't known Jackie was pregnant, when mutual friends Chris and Amy visited Vancouver from Minneapolis. "How did you pick your donor?" they asked. They were inseminating using a known donor, a friend of Chris's in Toronto, who'd had his sperm tested and frozen.

It was a good question. How do you pick a donor? If you have children the more traditional way, it's not something you're necessarily conscious of doing: choosing genetic material. And here we had a catalogue.

There were a couple of limiting factors. One was a blood-type thing: we needed someone who was Rh positive. The other was that we wanted a donor who would be willing to be known to the offspring (were the law to allow it) at age of majority. And, preferably, a donor who, if contacted by the offspring, would not freak out that the kid had been raised by lesbians. This ruled out Xytex, a sperm bank in the southern U.S. favoured by the fertility clinic we went to. We'd go through their catalogue and find a likely candidate, only to discover at the end of his pro-file that he was a member of the Promise Keepers (a kind of husbands-of-Stepford-wives Christian men's group). So we opted for Repromed, a sperm bank located in Toronto.

The Repromed catalogue tells you everything in one line: race, ethnicity, blood type, hair and eye colour, skin tone, height, weight, bone size, education and occupation, and interests. For example, Caucasian, Bulgarian, B positive, dark brown straight, green, medium olive, 5'8", 155 lb., small medium, Bachelor of Engineering, charity worker, hiking, soccer.

This sort of makes sense when you think that straight people using donor insemination are very often looking for a physical match for the husband. But what about us? We did not need a physical match. The question of race especially troubled us. Given that we're both white, something felt nastily white supremacist about choosing a white donor. And yet to choose a non-white donor felt reactive, like a political statement literally embodied in our child, who would then have to negotiate the repercussions of that choice (with help from us, naturally — but still). Neither option felt right. We debated closing our eyes and randomly stabbing at the page. Finally we fell back on the option of looking for someone like me, which at least gave us a starting point.

That's how we got Donor 3139, whom we promptly forgot about. Picking a donor seemed important only while we were doing it. Once the zygote was an embryo, it didn't matter.

"So what's the donor like?" asked Amy and Chris.

"Um, let me think. Dutch, tall, blue-eyed, easygoing, piano-teacher mother, parasitologist fa—"

"Hey, that sounds like Mary and Jackie's donor," said Chris, who is Mary's ex. Also my ex. The fact that we are all friends is very lesbian of us.

"Jackie's pregnant, did you know that?"

We didn't even know they were inseminating.

We had heard stories about this kind of thing: lesbians in Toronto whose kids were in preschool together noticing a resemblance and then discovering they'd used the same donor. We never imagined it would happen to us.

We wrote Mary and Jackie. Uh, did you by any chance use Donor 3139? Yes, in fact, they had.

Hoo. It *had* happened to us. What did this *mean*? A whole new meaning to "We are fa-mi-ly" at Gay Pride Day, but what else? We didn't really know.

DECEMBER 13, NO BABY. Cindy talks to the doctor. She has been going for an exam every couple of days. "If there's no baby after ten days," says the doctor, "we'll look at inducing."

Say I'd been playing Balderdash any time before Cindy got pregnant and someone said that a doula was (a) a Greek dish, (b) a Samoan fishing spear, or (c) a woman who aids in childbirth, I'd have gone with (a). Cindy would have liked to use a midwife, but all the midwives in Vancouver were booked. Every single one of 'em. Okay. Cindy liked her doctor, her doctor liked delivering babies. The doctor could deliver. "But maybe we should hire a doula for extra help." A what?

A doula is supposed to help with a range of non-medical birthing-type things—developing a birth plan; bringing the exercise ball to the delivery; offering a TENS machine (a neat device that provides alternative pain to distract you from the pain of childbirth, if I remember correctly); offering emotional support before, during, and after the birth; doing your laundry, should you need it; or making you a sandwich. Basically all the things I would've been doing. In fact, many times the doula we hired would take over the role I normally played in Cindy's life. I didn't get it. But what did I know about birthing babies? Nothing.

So we hired a doula. And in fact she gave us lots of information, like why not to immunize your baby and how many unnecessary Caesareans are performed in B.C. each year.

DECEMBER 14, NO BABY. December 15, no baby.

Seven weeks earlier, Cindy had crooned to her belly in a hotel room in Calgary. "Stay, little baby, stay. Don't come out now, baby. Just stay. The womb's a good place to be."

Eight months pregnant, she had hopped a plane from Vancouver after a call from the Banff Centre, where I'd been working. I'd been rushed by ambulance to Calgary with a high fever and a rampant internal infection unresponsive to antibiotics. The words *surgery* and *colostomy bag* were floating in the air above me as I lay semi-conscious. They were sounding pretty good.

"Oh, don't come out, don't come out. Little baby, stay in there, stay," she sang.

The baby, it seems, had listened.

DECEMBER 16. A CONTRACTION! A contraction? Yes, definitely something contracted. We wait. We watch the belly. It sits there, roundly. Not contracting. We wait some more. Nothing.

Oh. Braxton Hicks.

After two weeks in hospital in Calgary, I got the okay to come home to Vancouver. Five days later I was back in hospital. The only beds available were on the maternity ward, and I found myself in a room with a pregnant woman on complete bedrest and regular fetal monitoring, being visited by my very pregnant spouse. Pregnant lesbians are a matter of course at B.C. Women's Hospital, where they deliver practically every day. But pregnant lesbians visiting their nullipara spouses in the maternity ward at St. Paul's were a distinct oddity.

About a week after I was discharged for good—this would be late November—Cindy had a muscle spasm in the middle of the night that strained her Achilles tendon as badly as if, so the physiotherapist said, she'd run a marathon without training. So I was a pale, slowly recovering stick and she was using crutches or a wheelchair. Oh yeah, we were ready to be new parents.

DECEMBER 17. WE ARE ready. I've regained my strength and Cindy is walking unaided. The baby, however, is not ready. The baby is eleven days overdue. There is no sign of labour now, at the beginning of the period when it is riskier for the baby to stay in the womb than to be born. The doctor suggests trying the milder of the inducing options. So off we go to the hospital, drugs are injected—wait. Wait. Wait. Wait.

Wait.

By late afternoon there are still no contractions. Nothing. We go home.

DECEMBER 18. TWELVE DAYS overdue. Back to the hospital. Another exam, this time with the obstetrician as well as Cindy's doctor. There are no signs of impending labour—the baby's head has not dropped, the cervix is not ripe. And the baby's head is large. Very large. This is one of the factors that presents difficulties when pregnancy continues more than ten days past the due date. The baby is big and getting bigger. A big baby is harder to deliver. We could try oxytocin, but the family doctor and the obstetrician think that induced labour will end in a C-section anyway. That head just isn't going to fit through those hips, labour-induced muscle relaxing or no. We *could* wait another two days, but each day increases the chance of other complications. The baby could have its first poo, for example, which would float around in amniotic fluid and potentially be drawn into the baby's lungs, causing infection. Or the placenta could begin to degenerate, giving the baby less oxygen and fewer nutrients and reducing the amount of amniotic fluid.

When the doula learns the doctors are suggesting a Caesarean birth, what does she want to do? She wants to perform a ritual to help the baby withstand the trauma of coming into the world in such a violent, unnatural way.

"Get rid of her," Cindy says from her hospital bed. I get rid of the doula.

Some time before 4:00 p.m., Cindy is prepped for surgery, wheeled into the operating room, and moved onto the table. They set up a screen—a navy blue curtain about a foot high—across Cindy's chest. She can see the doctor's heads but not what they are doing. The anesthetist and I sit by her head. The anesthetist is very good at small talk, which handily serves to cover up the sound of the incision—a smooth *whssht*—followed by the snip of scissors through muscle. Do we know if it's a boy or a girl? the anesthetist asks. Do we have names picked out?

"Graeme," Cindy says. "Or Kate."

Cindy's doctor is young and about five feet tall. The obstetrician is old and about six foot three, a family friend of the young doctor. At first they chat idly about people they know, but quite soon they are pushing down on Cindy's belly. I realize they are going to squeeze the baby out, rather like squeezing toothpaste out of a tube.

"Push, Ally, push!" the old OB admonishes the doctor. The doctor gets up as high as she can and pushes down with all her weight and all her strength. Repeatedly. She grunts like a tennis player, *huhngh*, and then like a woman in labour, *aaaugherrrrrrrgh*. Apparently it's not easy to get a baby out of the womb any which way. A note of urgency enters the old guy's voice. "Put all you've got into it."

"I am," she says. A few tense moments. More pushing. More grunting.

And then? Squalling.

"You want to take a picture?" the OB says.

Picture? What? I've forgotten I have a camera in my hands. I stand, I point, but the flash is not ready. There's a baby coming out of that belly. A baby's head. Our baby's head.

"Hurry, hurry," he says.

I snap the picture, sans flash. The OB cradles the baby's head and slides the whole body out, clamps the umbilicus. A nurse hands me surgical scissors. The scissors seem to have a solemnity, a heft. It does not seem to be something that can be done quickly, cutting the cord, yet it must. Everyone in the operating room moves at a clip, everything is done swiftly, everyone moves with speed and assurance but me, caught in a time bubble, afraid to botch it, afraid to give this baby a lifelong weirdo innie or outie. I hold my breath. I snip.

The obstetrician holds her up for another picture. "You have a baby girl."

Cindy was convinced she was having a boy. Dream after dream after dream, the baby was a boy. Statistics suggested a boy: lesbians who conceive using frozen sperm have more boys than girls. But this is a girl. Kate, not Graeme.

Then the baby is being wiped clean, she's being weighed. I say something, I don't remember what, and the baby who listened so well in the womb turns her head towards me as if she recognizes the voice. Cindy says something next, and she turns her head again to the voice that sang, "Stay, my little baby. Stay safe and warm," and would now sing, "Welcome. Welcome to the world. All our troubles are over."

Six days later, also by Caesarean, Kate's half-sister, Clare, is born. My mother has recovered from both the pneumonia and the dementia and wants to be called Gran. My dad inadvertently calls himself Grandpa within twenty-four hours of seeing his tenth grandchild. "Have you got Grandpa's nose? Who's got Grandpa's nose?" The doula does our laundry, makes us a sandwich. Our troubles are not all over. No one's really are. But for a while it sure feels like it.

WINTER STAR

Peter Behrens

IT WAS WINTER ON the peninsula. February. The ground mostly bare. Some people were disappointed. They had anticipated the brightness, lightness, softness of snow.

But I like unconcealed ground. The clarity of brilliant days, of open frozen meadows sloping down to the sea. Their colour hard to describe. A kind of parched yellow, with a sheen of grey frost in early morning.

The powerful thing was the light returning, afternoons lengthening, and darkness gradually being pushed back. In a northern world there is nothing more hopeful. Days packed with light, packed with promise.

What I am trying to say is, the signs augured well. I don't know about the stars, don't know how to read stars, but the sun—the clarity and dazzle of those days in mid-winter—was encouraging.

BASHA HAD BEEN ON a shoot in Cincinnati when she started feeling pregnant. She never described the feeling exactly, but she badly wanted to come home. How she hated Cincinnati that week. Arriving home, she went straight upstairs to use a pregnancy test kit.

Birth experience, death experience. I had had more of the latter. My family had been shrinking for a long time, until it seemed defined by its losses. My father was dead. My sister Anne had been killed in a car wreck a few months before my mother died. Only my sister Mary and I were left, and neither of us had children.

Through the next nine months I tried to help Basha deal with the discomforts of her pregnancy, but didn't want to think a lot about my incipient fatherhood. I wasn't convinced it was incipient. It made me uncomfortable when Basha bought or was given baby clothes; such preparations seemed to be challenging fate a little too boldly. I was reluctant to help get a nursery room ready, didn't want to know the baby's sex. Sure, I had names in my head, boy names, girl names, but it made me uneasy to say them aloud. It seemed another unnecessary challenge to fate, which might be tempted to deliver a wicked backhand.

Most of this was undiscussed. I'd grown up in a vestigially Irish Catholic culture that was not in the habit of acknowledging its superstitions. Even talking about them could bring bad luck.

They did distract me from practical, reality-based worrying. How was I, an unpublished novelist, ever going to earn enough to support a family? Such mundane issues never troubled me, not for a second.

THE DAY IN FEBRUARY, roaring with light. Sunlight glowering across meadows, dashing off the blue sea.

In the morning, having tea with friends, Basha felt her water break. At least, she thought that was what had happened. The due date was still a week away. At noon she took herself for a blustery walk on High Street and felt a cramp, but it passed. Returning to the house, she telephoned Caroline, our doula.

We live eleven miles from the hospital. Caroline is two towns away from us. Her husband is an electrician, and they own a seafood restaurant on the wharf, open in summer. In winter Caroline volunteers to counsel pregnant mothers on the peninsula through the experience of childbirth. Doula is a strange new word, in our culture anyway, for someone in an ancient role, the mother's standby advocate, the wise woman. Caroline hopped in her Jeep and was at our house in half an hour. Together she and Basha decided that, yes, the water had definitely broken. Maybe the cramp had been early contractions, maybe not.

We had been attending new-parent classes at Blue Hill Hospital, along with sullen boys slouching uneasily, ball caps pulled low over their eyes, and teenage girls with anxious faces and strong Maine accents. They all looked about eighteen. Easily they could have been my children.

What I remembered from the classes:

Bundling is good.

Support the baby's head, because its neck muscles are weak.

Never use talcum powder: it gets in the lungs.

Don't bother coming to the hospital until you're getting contractions at twenty-minute intervals.

Caroline and Basha were in the kitchen. Basha was staring at an alarm clock brought down from our bedroom, when the set of contractions arrived, sharp and unmistakable. The interval had probably been an hour. No reason to go to the hospital. Not yet. We agreed that I might as well go for a run, and I went upstairs to change. When I came down, Basha was leaning over the kitchen counter, panting. There had just been another wave of contractions. Caroline was standing behind her, massaging her lower back.

Do you think I should go for a run? I said.

A fast one, Caroline said.

Basha started gasping.

How you feelin', hon? said Caroline.

Oh dear, said Basha.

Hurts, eh?

Yes. Oh. Oh. Oh.

Yep, said Caroline. Let's get mama to the hospital.

Uh, you mean after I run? I said.

No, now.

There followed the classic panicky drive to the hospital, me at the wheel and Basha gasping and writhing on a reclined front seat. It was the drive I had been anticipating—and looking forward to, I suppose—all my life. The roads were gritty with sand that had been spread on ice and snow that had long since melted. Basha was grunting with another flurry of contractions. I was driving too fast.

Still, I remember that road, the winter emptiness of it, yellow meadow grass in stiff bunches, that strong sunlight flaring on Blue Hill Bay. There were a couple of sharp bends on the Parker Point Road where I felt the front wheels starting to slide on the sand. Caroline, following us in the Jeep, had fallen behind, was out of sight.

Blue Hill Hospital is just old-fashioned enough that its suspicion of intrusive technology and pharmacology feels hip and contemporary. Very difficult pregnancies end up at Eastern Maine Medical in Bangor, an hour away; Blue Hill has a birthing tub. Basha, a swimmer and a sailor, had always liked the idea. Water is her beloved, familiar element. The nurses helped her climb into the tub. Her body was full and firm, like a not-quite-ripe peach. Caroline stood by. I began rubbing Basha's back and neck and shoulders, whenever the women let me get close enough. I was talking to her. Can't remember what I said. Probably trying to be funny.

Where I grew up, you try to make people laugh at the most painful, emotional moments. When things are scary. It's a way of renouncing, defying, or just avoiding reality. Also a technique for self-protection, for keeping your distance from undiagnosed emotions.

Another wave of contractions. Basha was squatting in the tub, gasping and shouting. More contractions. She said she was starting to feel cold. We helped her out of the tub. The women wrapped her in towels and guided her to a bed that cranked up into a seated position. She sat with her legs spread and the pain arriving in short, sharp shocks. She released it in little screeches, desperate whispers. After every screech she instinctively apologized to the nurses.

They were solid Maine women, amused by the apologies. You had the feeling that, like veteran non-coms, they had seen it all. Nothing was going to fluster them.

Women kept speaking to me over their shoulders, suggesting where I might stand to get the best possible camera angle when the baby came out. I was the only male in the room, and the only role open to me, apparently, was videographer. No one seemed to notice I didn't have a camera.

I should have been offended by the gender stereotyping, my assignment to passive observer status. Instead I felt we were both lucky, blessed even, that this powerful circle of women had gathered around Basha like a herd of Indian elephants and were guarding her ferociously.

I did, however, intend to get closer to the action. I kept sidling in, grabbing a hand, touching a shoulder, pushing back a strand of damp hair. She was riding waves of pain. It was terrifying to watch. I tried to gauge what the women were thinking. They didn't seem worried or tense, so everything was normal, presumably.

Then the baby was crowning. It was hard to believe that the white gleam of what looked like clean bone was the crown of our child's skull, trying to push its way out into the hospital world.

Push, push, push, the women were chanting.

After every sequence of pushes they allowed Basha a few moments to rest, then she had to start pushing again. They were ruthless. By now I had inserted myself into the bedside team and was allowed to support one of her legs. Our doctor, a shy young woman, new to the peninsula, had slipped into the room, but it was clear that the senior nurse was still in charge.

I was flushed with what might have been adrenalin. The only other time I remember feeling so charged was on a sub-zero afternoon when I fell through the ice on a lake in the Rockies. After floundering helplessly and nearly giving up, I managed to drag myself out of the hole, and as I flopped onto the ice I felt the adrenalin surging, delivering the jolt of strength and focus that I'd needed to survive the rest of that ordeal.

What it stimulated now was a fanatical instinct to protect Basha and our half-born baby. Protect them from what, exactly, I don't know. There was nothing threatening in that place. Nonetheless, all my hackles were up. If a stranger had bumbled into the room at that moment I might have flown at him and bitten his throat.

The cycle of pushing, short rest, and more pushing continued. The white skullcap was showing but nothing more. I saw the head nurse whisper something to the young doctor, who quietly assented. They were going to make a small vaginal incision. This was done quickly, and almost instantaneously the baby slipped out, packed in the shape of an egg, hugging itself within its own oval. I saw hormone-swollen testicles red as fire, and knew we had a son. Then the egg shape unfolded itself like a piece of origami. He waved his arms, kicked his legs, unscrunched his face, and immediately transmitted a sequence of expressions suggesting by turns resentment, confusion, fear, wonder, curiosity, and hunger. Each mood lasting for maybe a second. He let out a yowl. They were wiping him down, bundling him, putting a silly bright blue toque on his head, and handing him off to me while the doctor quickly sewed up his mother.

I carried the boy down the hospital corridor, hackles still up. His defender, protector, advocate, bodyguard. His father.

(Later I learned that my sister Mary, at that same hour, was flying over Montreal and looking down at the cemetery where our grandparents, aunts, uncles, cousins, parents, sister are buried. So life was a circle after all. A wheel that might keep spinning, not a dead end.)

The nurse led us into a bright room, where she briskly weighed, measured, injected. I carried the boy back to Basha and her mother, who had just arrived. I could feel my parents stir in the ground. I could imagine my sister Anne's laughter.

Himself nursed greedily. Then Basha nibbled bland hospital food while the boy's grandmother and I took turns holding him. Suddenly famished, I headed off to the local roadhouse bar to grab a hamburger and a glass of beer. When I returned, he was feeding again. When he was done, I lay back in a faux-leather reclining chair with him on my chest. The weight of him containing the future.

They were asleep when I left. I'd promised to come back first thing in the morning, bringing Basha a latte from the Blue Hill Co-op and a bagel with smoked salmon and cream cheese.

Black loam sky above the hospital parking lot, jabbed with stars.

I drove along the coast road with all windows cranked down, the winter scent of balsam and fir floating through the car, and the sharp, complex aroma of the sea. As soon as I got home I dug out a framed photograph of my grandfather, who had died before I was born, and whom our son was named after. Then I put on a CD of Bach's cello suites and turned the volume up loud. I felt like a kind of animal, crudely and deeply satisfied, and with the violent music roaring through the house, I went upstairs to bed and to sleep.

FIVE TIMES

Kathy Page

IT'S STILL DARK, 5:45 a.m., but a rush of footsteps wakes me a moment before the gasp of cold air. You lift the covers and climb into our bed, your chilled bare skin relaxing into supernatural smoothness.

"You're warm!"

"Ssh. Sleep."

Head under my chin, you stretch, squirm, turn, turn again, then turn the other way, elbow my belly, thrust your icy buttocks into my bladder. You sigh, wait three seconds, corkscrew yourself up the bed until your static-shocked hair tickles my nose and your breath blows hot and damp onto my neck. I feel the beginning of your laughter as your left hand creeps towards my armpit, and I squeeze tight, trapping it, then spread my hand across your back.

"Can you stay still, sweetheart?"

"Like this?" You freeze, every muscle taut, fists clenched, belly, knees, and ankles rigid: an almost six-year-old boy less than a metre long. Then you melt and sit up, pulling the covers away as you do.

"I'm too awake!"

Beside me, Richard groans, turns, digs deeper into his dream, and then your eyes light on my nipples, erect in the cold; you pull the shirt up for a better look. We both know where this will lead: you'll run your finger along our scar, the thin thread of white that runs just north of my pubic hair (a few days ago you pointed out a grey one, but it's gone now).

"Here," you'll say, looking into my eyes for confirmation. "That's where I came out... *not* here," you say, pointing between my legs.

"Yes, you came out that way. It didn't hurt."

"Let's play," you say. *"Please. Let's play me being born."* We've played this game for years now, countless times, all possible ways. Today you choose the kind of birth where I'm caught completely by surprise. I think it's gas or overeating. I think I might call the doctor, but then — ouch! — you shoot out, announce your own name, and proceed to outline in broken English your unwillingness to sleep in a crib and a preference for chocolate milk.

———

"YOU OKAY?" ANITA ASKS. We met for the first time three or four hours ago; she's the midwife on duty tonight, a tiny, olive-skinned woman with soft brown eyes and cool hands. She frowns, studies my face. She says she definitely wants a doctor's opinion, and a few enormous minutes or maybe a short hour later he arrives — very tall, very young. Pink skin, loud voice. He reaches out a well-scrubbed hand, and in order to grasp it I have to release one of my own hands from the padded bench I'm clutching.

"Dr. Ryan," he says.

"Kathy."

"Richard."

These introductions seem oddly formal under the circumstances. While we speak, it seems as if someone is just now tightening spiked metal bands around my lower half. The whole damn thing may be natural, but it is also pretty strange. Who could even dream it up?

Distraction—jokes, wordplay, mind games—is what works for me, and Richard is my accomplice (*police, pace, lice, limp, come*). I'm not sure that Anita approves.

Dr. Ryan studies the file Anita has handed him, a document called the "Pre-birth Statement." Last time, I remember, the same piece of paper was called the "Birth Plan."

"Forty-two. Second baby. Prefers minimal intervention," he reads aloud, frowning as if he has difficulty making out the words. "Yes?" he asks, as another contraction (*tract, contract, iron, rant, rain, action, train*), this one a wave with teeth, breaks in my flesh. Richard kneads my back, but it's as if I'm two people—or if I count you inside me trying to get out, three—and the backrub is happening to one of the others.

Where were we?

Intervention (*invent, intent, rent, vent, nerve, Triton*) and how we all want to avoid it. We've talked to our mothers, read studies. Everyone yearns for the home birth I almost had with Becky: two intense days of labour, then an exhausted but hilarious dash to the hospital; gulping down gas until the tank was dry; finally, the bliss of anesthesia.

"But there was no tearing at all, and I did avoid the forceps," I am telling Dr. Ryan when a contraction comes again, tightening, spreading. Think (*thin, ink, kin, hit*)? Speak (*peas, asp, peak*)? No (*on*).

And then it passes.

"I'm not a fanatic," I explain. "We've come to the hospital. I'm not squatting in the woods. But just, you know—"

"Yes," he says, turning away. "So, Anita, she's seven centimetres dilated, and this one is posterior too. Her waters should have broken by now...I'd like to break them." He turns back to me. "It's a simple thing, hardly what you'd call an intervention. Might get things going."

It's the slippery slope, Helen from prenatal yoga would say, but it's also a matter of timing: the spiked wave/belt is at its tightest, so I say yes and then think, *Sorry*, because maybe you're just not quite perfectly ready and we're all being impatient. However, I'm not sure how long I can continue this way.

Time shrinks, stretches, and bends, grows shorter and wider at the same time. I sit, wait for the contraction, swing legs, wait, open legs apart, wait. I let Anita tip me back the correct amount, then wait for Dr. Ryan to prepare.

"My wife said no intervention, but she lasted about half an hour," he informs us as he pulls on some milky white rubber gloves (*slobber, glob, love*). Richard squeezes my shoulder.

"I'll wait till this one's over," Dr. Ryan says, and then his hand disappears. There's just an arm and a view of the top of his head, the hair, thick and dull blond, systematically cut. A jostling in the cunt.

"Nothing there," he says. "Your waters have broken already." Nothing there?

Spiked wave. Metal band. Belt of blades. Whatever it is tightens again and a vast herd of horses with knived hooves gallops over my back, even though I'm lying on it—don't expect logic (*Log, go, I*).

"Are you sure you don't remember anything?"

It feels wrong to be on my back, but I can't speak to tell them. Someone drills a hole in my sacrum. Anita reminds me to breathe. I throw up.

"I'd like to introduce a scalp monitor," Dr. Ryan says.

"Is there a problem?"

"Your baby has a heightened risk of infection because of the lack of amniotic fluid."

"It's okay. Everything will be okay," Anita reassures us as Dr. Ryan's face disappears again.

Now we can see your heart rate dip with every contraction. "It's normal for the heartbeat to slow down a little during a contraction and then pick up."

"Is this a little?"

"We'll keep watching. Have you given him a name yet?"

"James."

"Owen," Richard and I say in almost unison. A dozen heartbeats pass, and in the room next door a woman screams. Not once but continuously, pausing only for breath — gulp after gulp of air, scream after scream, stuck in a crescendo that never peaks.

"Well," Anita says to Dr. Ryan, "that's Mrs. Sovak letting everyone know." A mixture of acid and glass splinters, introduced through the hole in my lower back, forces its way through capillaries, shreds them, gathers where your head must be.

Mrs. Sovak screams on.

"Look," Dr. Ryan says, "it's absolute chaos in Maternity tonight. There's nothing worse than wanting anesthesia and having to wait in line. I'm going to order you an epidural. If you don't want it, you can send it away when it arrives."

Am I ready for this? Do I like Dr. Ryan? I can't tell, because Mrs. Sovak's screams have carved out the last bit of my brain.

"Consent," the form is headed. I don't read it because I already know: for you, increased risk of feeding problems, inconsolability, slower bonding in the first six weeks; for me, even slower labour and further intervention, fever, back trauma, headache, paralysis.

But it was fine last time.

I sign, and then, as if the two events were connected, the screaming next door stops. Has Mrs. Sovak delivered her baby? I want to be told, "Yes! It's lying on her stomach right now," but neither Anita nor Dr. Ryan replies.

We watch your heart rate dip and rise. "Don't worry," Anita repeats (and don't think about waves, belts, horses, knives, drills). And don't look at the clock. But do breathe (*hate, heat, breath, heart, hearth, rate, tear*), which is supposed to relax you but actually intensifies the pain. Do they tell you to breathe so that you remind yourself you are alive, that there are two things, you and the pain, and you're still there?

No, dummy, it's so the baby gets enough oxygen. Oxygen in, carbon dioxide out. What about those other gases in the air? What are they? Remember physics with Mr. Porter, who got Penny Barker pregnant? Nitrogen. Helium. Hydrogen. Xenon? Argon? Moron? Neon? Why don't we glow?

"Are you all right?"

A short man wearing a neat turban and rimless spectacles has materialized near my head.

Do I want the epidural? Yes (*yes*).

"Excuse me," the anesthetist says as the needle goes in, and minutes later, the pain is wiped away.

Richard takes my hand in his and it's like I'm coming back to earth: I see, now, how tired Richard looks, how tiny Anita is, how her face is a perfect oval, that Dr. Ryan is very tall indeed and his shoulders slump forwards, that the little anesthetist has lovely hands, immaculate nails. And that containing us all is this cream-painted room, a cheerful print of daffodils hung lonely but brave in the middle of the only wall not occupied by equipment, shelves, or furniture.

I'm lying on my side now, watching the monitor, where I see your heart rate dip, then rise.

Dr. Ryan twitches a smile and props himself against the shiny steel sink unit, arms folded across his chest.

"I'd like to lay out some options," he says as your heart rate dips again. "You haven't progressed in the past six hours, and we don't know why. There was no amniotic fluid for we don't know how long. There's distress — acceptable at this point and level, but not if it gets worse or continues for a long time. Then we're looking at a C-section."

"Continues how long?" Richard asks as your heart rate recovers.

"It depends," Dr. Ryan says, "on the whole picture. We have to play it by ear." It dips.

"But is there a risk in waiting?" Rises.

"We're monitoring. So at any point—" Dips.

"Look," I say, "let's just do it now."

"Yes," says Dr. Ryan, without a pause or a blink, "I think that's best. I'll call through to theatre."

Theatre (sounds like *they ate 'er*): a hot place with intense, super-white light beamed down from above. The screen across my chest saves us from seeing what they do, but we hear every-thing: the way Dr. Ryan breathes out through his teeth, the tinkle of an instrument he's handed to his assistant to discard. And I can feel—not pain—but something: shifts of pressure, movement. I can no longer see the monitor and wish I could, but I know to be calm, not to dwell on what can't be, or on this being an *emergency*, or on your distress, or that it's absolutely down to Dr. Ryan now, how we come out of this.

"Is this good?" the anesthetist asks.

"Fantastic," I tell him, and I tell you that we'll be all right: this has happened before. From the start of the surgery it will be about fifteen minutes until you're delivered. The rest of it is just sewing up. That's what Dr. Ryan said.

"*Theatre* contains," I tell Richard, looking into his lovely eyes and ignoring that he looks, as I must, totally demented. "*Theatre* contains *rate, rat, that, threat, treat, heat, heath, tree, three*—" and somehow I've got myself into Macbeth, where I don't want to be.

"Shall I tell you," he suggests, "about the new bathroom we're going to have?" *Root, moat, brat, mat, bar.*

"Go ahead."

"New shower, obviously. I thought brushed metal, because it's not so harsh. Then some white tiling, four-inch, but with a band of mosaic in earth tones..."

"Roman-looking?"

"Yes. Same behind the bath. Softer lighting."

"What about the floor?" I ask, and see Richard's eyes mimic mine, startle wider, because on the other side of the screen that bisects me, Dr. Ryan has put his hands inside my womb to take you out. I can feel them.

"Floor?" Richard says, slowly. The word is meaningless, but we cling to it. "Floor. Well, I think it should be a heated floor." A painless cataclysm unfolds in my womb, and then I feel only absence. There's a moment of complete silence at the other end of me. Then Dr. Ryan says, "Here he is!" and I love the man not just for what he's done but for the catch in his voice. "Get that cord off his neck," he says. "Looks like a multiple. One," he says, "two...three." His voice rises. "Four...*five*. Good God, he had the cord around his neck *five times*..."

"Is he all right?"

No one answers. Five times. No wonder, they're all saying. Five times!

"Is he all right?"

There's a faint, half-animal wail, and Richard and I are kissing the tears from each other's faces.

"Seems fine," Dr. Ryan's voice informs us. There's an edge of disbelief to it. "Bit of meconium. Getting washed and doing his tests. Has to go to ECU, but you can hold him first..."

Something else happens inside. Dr. Ryan breathes out through his teeth.

"I'm closing up your uterus now."

"Where's my baby?"

There at last you are, on my chest and in my hands: bald, huge-headed, your eyes squeezed tight against the light, your skin bright purple-pink against the white blanket. Hello, hello, hello...How far you've come for this first meeting, and yet you're still travelling on, farther into unknown territories, breath after breath, eyes closed, hands tightly curled. By the time Dr. Ryan appears from behind the screen, you're sucking hard and beginning to relax.

We blurt out our thanks. And when we're done, he waits, makes sure both of us have torn our eyes away from you.

"That was a good decision," he says, and these words, spare as they are, manage somehow to convey that the four of us — midwife, doctor, mother, and father — made the good decision just in time.

It's the oddest kind of intimacy, this: to have your child's life and your own saved by someone you've barely met, who stands there now, exhausted, ready to go off shift and back home.

We shake hands again.

His clogs, I notice as he walks out of our lives, are covered in my blood.

THREE THOUSAND, FOUR HUNDRED AND FIFTY

Christine Pountney

IT'S HARD TO WRITE when you're this tired, when you're this obliterated by love, when you have fallen into the pools of your own son's deep blue eyes.

He's asleep in the other room. He's only six weeks old and yet he could be a million years old. I don't know where he's from. I can't tell. Another planet. He is gorgeous. His breath, I can't get over it. His skin is so luminous. The gentle, tender movements of his hands. The way he communicates with his fingers. The warm, downy roundness of his head. The way he reclines in the big metal salad bowl I use to bathe him, like an old man in a hot tub. The slow blink. The face that keeps saying, What? What? The sounds he makes when he's breastfeeding, like he's eating porridge with a wooden spoon out of a wooden bowl. I keep thinking how anthropomorphic he is and then have to remind myself that he is already human. Then, so adult-like. That look he has, like he's forcing himself to be patient. His expressions are so extreme I wonder if they are matched on the inside by feelings equally extreme. I try to put a name to them. Perplexed astonishment. Dubious alarm. A weary stoicism. Recently, elation, in the form of a smile.

At the beginning I kept crying for love of him and because the world scares me sometimes. My horoscope recommended visualizing mud and an old shoe being pulled from my body in a ritual act of healing. I have him in bed with me at night, then fall asleep and dream that one of his hands has fallen off like the head of a rose, and wake up with a start and he's still sucking on my breast. Or I'll wake up and look frantically for him, patting the soft humps of duvet before realizing that his father is walking him up and down the hall. So strange, this waking-sleeping limbo. All I know for certain is that I love him. It's so amorous, this feeling, and so sensual. I keep kissing his face. I can smell him on me when he's not around. And his little voice. I feel I know him and yet I don't really know what that means. He's so indistinct or undefined and yet fully himself — and I know who that self is, but it's more like holding a texture or a colour or a warmth.

The baby's father is on a cross-country book tour while I'm at home in my housecoat. I breastfeed and feel invisible while he gets congratulated for being a parent. His career has been forced into overdrive by new feelings of responsibility, while mine is receding like the caboose on a train that is barrelling away from me. This is a new dynamic, and sometimes I feel overwhelmed and resent all the woman-work I'm doing. The rest of the time I stare into my baby's eyes like a love-struck teenager and shiver with pleasure.

His eyes. They are as big as they will ever be. Sometimes, when I stare at them long enough, they look like the eyes of a thirty-five-year-old. My own age.

His existence in the world may be miraculous, but it is irreversible now. His origins may be inexplicable — where was he before he existed? — but his presence now is so obvious. He is so real, so irrevocable. The whole person is already there, his disappearance unimaginable. How did the world ever exist without him?

I am not selfless. I don't want to be selfless. And yet I am better to him than I have ever been to anyone. My desires are shelved — my impatience and my ambition. They are denuded the moment he looks at me, the moment he needs something from me. This is an obliterating love. Did I already use the word *obliterating*?

The daze. The putting of the milk in the cupboard and the honey in the fridge. Already I am forgetting what he looked like as a newborn. I will forget what he looks like now. What this feels like. What it felt like to give birth. I am too shattered to retain these things. I'm still close enough to the birth to remember the outline of it, the bulky shape like an imposing figure in a black cowl looming in the corner of every room, but it is fading. I can actually feel the pull of my memories receding. They are waving from the caboose of that train barrelling down the tracks away from me. Before it disappears entirely from sight, I must try to remember what it was like. What was it like to give birth?

Let me just say that pregnancy does not prepare you. Pregnancy by comparison is a honeymoon.

I found out I was pregnant at the Toronto Catholic District School Board headquarters. I was there for an interview, to teach creative writing to high-school students, and fifteen minutes early. I had a pregnancy test in my purse that I'd bought earlier in the day because my period was late and my boyfriend and I were trying. I didn't think I was pregnant but I thought, what the hell, because I'd seen four teenage girls walk down the hall in short

kilts and white shirts and plaid ties and the sight of them triggered an old feisty sense of rebellion I can't seem to suppress even
at this age. I am not obedient; I have a problem with authority.
I thought, I'll do the test and then leave it on the floor of the
bathroom stall and see if that spreads chaos among the nuns.
I'm not even sure they have nuns at the TCDSB, but they did in
my day when I attended an all-girls Catholic school in Montreal
for three years before they kicked me out.

So I did the test. I put the stick on the chrome toilet paper
dispenser. I stood up from a crouch and zipped up my jeans. Was
that a pink line slowly appearing? I held the stick up and twisted
it under the poor fluorescent lighting. I walked out to the sinks
and held it to the mirror and saw it in reflection. The pink strip
was deepening like a blush. So often I had imagined a little boy
appearing at the bedroom door in the middle of the night, and
lifting my head and then the sheet to let him crawl into bed
beside me. But here I was at the starting line of an experience
I could barely imagine, let alone control. In an instant the issue
of pregnancy went from being a question about me and what
I wanted to the introduction of another person on the scene
and what I could do, and would have to do, for them. I could no
longer think of being a parent in the same indulgent way. Hope
is so reckless it can actually catapult you ahead of the incident
you are wishing for so you can practise feeling nostalgic about
it. I put the test gingerly back into its box and left the bathroom.
The next time I looked up from the floor it was to say yes to my
new employer when he cheerfully asked, "Are you ready?"

The pregnancy was good news. It was planned, it was anticipated. It happened sooner than we'd thought. I told my boyfriend
in the kitchen and without ceremony. I don't have the patience for
ceremony and am incapable of delaying gratification, although

I did manage to say, "I want you to remember this moment," before blurting out that he was going to be a father.

I had been to Montreal for ten days just before this announcement and had drunk a lot of red wine and insisted on going to Au Pied de Cochon when none of my friends wanted to go, for foie gras and duck breast out of a can. The only reservation I could secure on short notice was for 5:30 on a Friday evening, so I arrived, the very first patron, and ate my meal alone at the bar while watching the sous-chefs set up large cauldrons of boiling water and braise pigs' trotters on the open grill. I figured—after tackling the predictable puritan anxiety to the ground—that it was good for the baby to have had a taste of decadence in preparation for the long months of deprivation that lay ahead. I would not drink again for the duration of my pregnancy, except for the last month, when an occasional glass seemed right and felt well deserved.

I was healthy and in good shape. I went swimming once a week and started attending yoga classes at my local YMCA, led by a diminutive Indian man of indeterminate age who would say, in a thick accent that seemed to float down from a high register like a leaf falling off a tree, "And now, good friends, prepare yourself for the relaxation of this position."

Six weeks later I was in Havana, weaving a moped through heavy diesel traffic, buzzing down a tree-lined driveway to look at Ernest Hemingway's house. At seven months I flew to London to visit a wealthy friend. She took me to a really fancy yoga studio, where I attended an official maternity class with one other woman and the instructor. This woman had just come back from Italy, where she had done yoga on Sting's sprawling Tuscan estate. The instructor led us through the toughest, most satisfying yoga class I've ever taken, one specifically tailored for preparing the body for birth. Halfway through I was lying on my back with my legs in the air and holding the soles of my feet, in the happy baby pose, and squeezing, as per her instructions, first my clitoris, then my vagina, and lastly my anus. How intimate the conspiracy of wealth allows the rich to be.

By June I was eight months pregnant and my boyfriend and I had relocated from Toronto to a hundred-year-old derelict house we own in Newfoundland, which we bought for a song and have been fixing up. It has no running water and there was still a lot of work to do to make it comfortable for the two of us, let alone a newborn.

All of this is to say I went in cocky. I thought birth would be a breeze. My mom had had short labours and small babies. My friends thought it would be a cinch for me. I wasn't fazed. I had been accident-prone as a child, had broken bones and crashed a motorcycle. I thought I had a high pain threshold. I knew it was going to be emotional—I was the only person in the prenatal class to sob at the videos of other women giving birth—but I was looking forward to the intensity.

There was a snag, however. Our plans to have the baby in the small rural hospital near our house were thwarted when the OB-GYN we liked told us she would be returning home to the mango plantation where she had grown up in India for the two weeks before and after my due date. The first locum to replace her was an immigrant doctor from Ghana. He confirmed that I was still only one centimetre dilated a few days before my due date. I asked him if he knew approximately how big the baby would be and he looked pleased to have been asked, even rubbing his hands together in delight. He said, "Well, this is not scientific," and put his hands on my belly and felt it from all sides while staring at the wall in concentration, "but I'm fairly good at this." Then he said, "Three thousand, four hundred and fifty."

My boyfriend and I both laughed out loud. We'd never heard such a large number in relation to a baby before, or one as specific as that. "Grams," the doctor said, then he laughed too, which I thought was a good sign, but the baby still hadn't arrived by the time he left and another locum arrived to replace him.

I first laid eyes on this new OB-GYN as he followed a miserable teenage girl out of his office. He looked to be of retirement age. His shoulders were stooped. He had a hooked nose and half-moon glasses connected to a silver chain that hung around his neck. He was the Grinch who stole Christmas. He was the teacher from *The Wall*. He was my worst nightmare and I hadn't even met him yet. My boyfriend sensed my repulsion and put his hand on my thigh. I watched the teenager sidle up to her mother, who was wearing a shiny purple tracksuit and hot-pink Crocs and was already primed for the outdoors with a fresh unlit cigarette. The girl skulked out of the office and I wanted to skulk out behind her.

There are some gynecologists who ought to be gynecologists and there are some who ought to do other things. This man had no bedside manner. He did not inspire confidence. In the examining room he seemed oblivious to the protocol surrounding my undressing. As he spoke to my boyfriend, he rested his hands on me as if I were a cut of beef and he a butcher giving advice on how best to prepare and roast me.

I consider myself a feminist, especially with regard to the rights I have over my body. So it dismayed me to think I might not be comfortable with or able to choose the conditions surrounding my own birthing experience. I did not like that the maternity ward in this hospital was named after a man. I hated the idea that Braxton Hicks contractions are named after the man who so-called discovered them. The bottom line for me was that, in the event of complications, this awkward OB-GYN was the person who would take a scalpel to my belly. It wasn't a personal thing, but I did not feel confident in his abilities.

That night I wrestled over the decision to go to St. John's, where we had no history or doctor or even accommodation. We had offers from friends, but when you're past your due date and waiting around for the first viable contraction, the last thing you want to be is a guest. It would mean a hotel room, for as many nights as it took before I went into labour. I was two days overdue already. I felt anxious. I felt enormous and uncomfortable. My baby was past the 3,450-gram mark and growing.

I was worried about what people would think. Would I seem a prima donna to demand a transfer at the last minute? I called my sister and she said, "This is your experience. You have every right to demand whatever it is that will make you feel comfortable."

I said, "If there was nobody else but me, if I was all on my own, I would go to St. John's."

"Then that is what you have to do."

I told my boyfriend and he called a hotel and booked us a room. Now that the threat of having to rely on that locum had passed, my repulsion for him turned to compassion, and I wondered what manner of sorrows had occurred in his life to leave him so socially disconnected.

We spent three nights in a St. John's hotel. We had running water and cable TV. We walked around Signal Hill in the bright sun. It was like Club Med. We scrambled to find an OB-GYN and were referred to a Dr. Kum. He was a chubby Asian man with such a reassuring bedside manner I hardly even noticed the student doctor he introduced, and had examine my cervix first, when normally I bristle at being anybody's textbook. I was five days past my due date and still only one centimetre dilated. Dr. Kum examined me next and gave me the royal root, which is a kind of swirling stretch of the cervix with the finger. It hurt, but I was so relieved to be in the hands of someone I could trust that I laughed it off. I sat up joking, all smiles. Funny how you can feel so reassured by someone almost at first sight. Dr. Kum was discreet. At my jokes he allowed a small lift at the corner of his mouth. He was aloof and yet warm. He was responsive. He listened where the other doctor had rambled on in a bumbling way. You only had to tell Dr. Kum anything once and he would get it. He was good at what he did. It made sense that he was in the business of delivering babies. I wanted to hug him. Had he let me, I would probably have cried. Something monumental was in the air, something at once incredibly common and incredibly miraculous. It's hard to get away from that word — miraculous — when you're trying to describe what it's like to have a baby.

The following evening we went out for sushi. I hadn't had sushi in nine months. It tasted delicious. We watched a movie on TV and fell asleep. Every minute of the day was now distracted by waiting. Every movement or kick or twinge was a possible: Is this it? I was beginning to resign myself to an induction. I was dreaming a lot. I woke up at 5:30 a.m. with a pain, like a muscle tensing, and then it passed. I lay in bed. Eight minutes later, another tensing pain. I got up and went to the bathroom. I thought, this is it. Or was it? I had a bath. I paced. It was definitely coming in a rhythm of every eight minutes. I sat down on the other double bed and put my hand on my boyfriend's shoulder.

"Babe," I said. "Babe."

He rolled over.

"I think I'm in labour."

"Aw, baby," he said, as if I'd just won a raffle or a door prize. "That's great." Then he rolled over again and went back to sleep.

I paced for another half-hour. I was beginning to sweat with nervousness.

"Babe." I shook him again, more forcefully. "I think we have to go the hospital. Right now."

When he has to get up, my boyfriend can be up in two seconds flat, standing with his knees bent and his hands out, looking as if someone's about to throw him something he desperately needs to catch.

Like maybe a baby.

We drove to the hospital. My boyfriend had made, that very morning, the front cover of the books section of the *Globe and Mail*, so I read the review out loud as he drove. We took the elevator up to the case room and they sent me to triage. I wanted someone to come and see me right away. The pain was already pretty overwhelming. It was deep, like it was emanating from the marrow of my bones, small bones in my armpits and wrists and the backs of my knees. Bones like thorns that shot out like claws. I thought, I'm gonna have this baby any minute. The staff was in the middle of a shift change. A nurse said, "Someone will be here in a minute. Walk around if it makes you feel better."

"I need an IV," I said. "I've got a heart murmur."

"Someone will be with you in a minute," she repeated and left in a hurry.

"Do you have the birth plan?"

My boyfriend whisked it out. It was handwritten, with a cartoon strip he'd drawn of a bear crawling into a cave and then re-emerging with a bear cub in its arms. I'd said, "You wish," when he showed it to me. We had a list of the things I did not want. I did not want an epidural. I did not want an episiotomy.

I stood up and held on to my boyfriend, and we strolled out into the ward. There was a loop of the hall you could do. Every six minutes or so I would double over in pain. I heard a woman giving birth. Every moan would end in a scream. A voice shouted, "That's it, that's it. Push. You're doing it. That's excellent. Keep pushing." We passed another couple in the hall, a younger couple. She was in a hospital gown. He was in brown wool and denim. They were shuffling too. She was holding on to a rail screwed to the wall, and bending forward. We looked like two old women in a retirement home being visited by their sons. I smiled but she didn't smile back. That scared me.

Back in triage, a doctor inspected my vagina. Everything sore. The bloody show. I was given a maxi pad and told to go for a walk.

What?

"Just for a couple of hours. Go out for breakfast and then come back. You're not officially in labour yet. You're only two centimetres dilated, and we like at least three or four. So we're not going to admit you just yet."

I'm not in labour? And it's this painful already? I could almost hear the wind go out of my sails. I had to regroup. I needed a new strategy. This was going to be much harder than I thought.

We got as far as the parking lot, then I said, "I have to go back. I'm in too much pain."

In the elevator an older woman said she'd been there herself and wasn't it wonderful and didn't she know what I was going through. I was clutching the side of the elevator and squeezing my boyfriend's sleeve. If she knew, then why the fuck didn't she stop talking?

On my return I was mercifully admitted, given an IV and a room, and shown to the ensuite bathroom, where I could get in the shower. I was shivering and weak. It was only 8:30 in the morning and all my energy had drained out of me. I sat down on a stool in the bathtub while my boyfriend held the shower head to the back of my neck. I was as slumped and spineless as if I had been dropped onto that stool from a great height. It was at this point that my eyes closed. It was like my body had drawn the curtains. I was battening down the hatches, retreating into myself for the storm that lay ahead. I would not open my eyes again until the baby was born. I would also not swear, except for once, and I would not speak to my boyfriend except to ask him to remove his watch.

The pain was coming from an area of my body I didn't know I had. I realized I had a basement, and that's where the pain was coming from. It was cold and damp. I began to understand that this ordeal would require every kilojoule of energy I possessed, and I could not afford to waste even the slightest effort on what wasn't essential. I shrunk down into a kind of asceticism; I can't call it discipline because I had no choice. The same paring down happened in my mind as well. Feelings I would normally indulge in were dismissed — anger, defiance, rebellion, indignation. I was in survival mode and it consisted of a stark nothingness, like an empty cement cell in which I stood naked, facing the pain, which was like a vapour or an invisible mist that would engulf and suffocate me and then pass, leaving me shivering and soaked and waiting for the next surge. My friend had described her labour as a wave that would toss her onto the shore, drag her out again, then toss her back onto the beach. It was that kind of exhausting pummelling, like a severe and ruthless beating.

It was still early on and I understood that my cervix was being sluggish — it wasn't ripe, it wasn't dilating — and I went through a period of disappointment in myself. I thought, You've gone and got yourself pregnant and thought in your cocky way that you could do this. There was some comfort in admitting that I couldn't do this, even when I knew there was no alternative.

There was a moment when I thought, I hate this. I simply hate this. But it was a hatred so impassive there were no histrionics. It was a hatred that had no power over the thing it hated, so it was almost a cheerful hatred, it was that matter-of-fact.

It was at this demoralizing point that I was told to move back to the bed by a nurse whose voice I didn't recognize. I could barely move. She said, "Okay, Christine, you have to move." This is when I swore. I opened my eyes and puked into the bidet. It was bright green, the colour of lime peel. My eyelids slammed shut again.

It wasn't until after the birth that I realized the nurse I had had up to this point and loved with all my heart was on a break. I had no conception of time. I didn't know that four hours had gone by. I couldn't understand where she could be. How many times had I transferred from the bed to the shower and back again? When I lay down this time, I couldn't imagine ever getting up again. With every contraction I cycled my legs under the sheets, violently, as if I were trying to run somewhere, like in those nightmares when you run and go nowhere or you run too slowly. I sat up and hoisted myself onto my knuckles and hung there. My favourite nurse returned. I heard her voice. There was talk of an epidural. I did not want an epidural. In my mind an epidural was as likely to kill me as this. I could have a shot of Demerol. *Demerol?* I thought. Where was the nurse? She had left again. I opened my eyes long enough to locate my boyfriend.

"Get the nurse," I seethed. "And get me that shot of Demerol, now!"

The contractions were speeding up, so they had to time the injection right.

"Don't move," someone said, then a needle bit into the flesh of my buttocks.

I felt buffeted and battered, like a ship breaking apart on the rocks. I didn't realize I was in the transition phase. The nurse was checking my cervix again.

"That's excellent, Christine. You're almost ten centimetres now. You've gone from eight to ten really quickly. Things are speeding up. I think we're gonna have this baby."

That was a surprise. I'd almost forgotten the purpose of this agony. *A baby?* I thought. *A baby?* The word warmed me, it melted me a little, or maybe it was the Demerol. Between contractions I expired like a Victorian. If my eyes had been open I would have been staring at the back of my wrist. I would sigh, just the once, and another contraction would be upon me like a savage dog ripping at my throat. I wanted to cry. It was too soon. I wasn't ready for another one.

"Okay," I heard the nurse say. "I want you to look at me, Christine."

The nurse was younger than me. She was pretty. "I can see the baby's head."

"What?"

"I need you to work with me now. You're not doing yourself any favours by making all this noise. When you feel a contraction, I want you to breathe, okay? Is that another one?"

I nodded like a child.

"Okay, breathe out. Push all the air out."

It's true, the breathing helped. It was better than yelling.

That contraction passed. The nurse was all business now. Her voice had changed.

"When I tell you to push, Christine, I want you to push. Do you understand me?"

I nodded again. I was putty in her hands. Did I tell you that I loved her? I was all hers. She was my mom. She was wiping the snot off my face and tying my shoe. I wanted to curl up in her lap, because that savage dog was galloping towards me again, strings of saliva whipping around his teeth. His feet left the ground, he was soaring towards me.

"Do you have the urge to push?" I did.

"So push!" she shouted. And I did. "And now stop."

"But I can't!"

"Don't push," someone said.

There were doctors in the room. Three doctors. A bright light. A young man in green scrubs was sitting between my knees. The same young man who had come in earlier to break my waters. Who had begun to tell me the risks involved, that it could lead to a Caesarean. My boyfriend had said, "I don't think she needs to hear this right now," and in my ascetic state, my saintly efficiency, I had interrupted to say, "That's okay. He has to tell me this."

It was in this state of mind that I had also accepted, without protest, that Dr. Kum was not on duty and a doctor I had never met before would be delivering my baby. As it turned out, a junior doctor overseen by a senior doctor—it was a teaching hospital and so far everyone had been excellent. I was in good hands. I trusted the executive decision. And besides, the head was coming. There was some hope now, jumping out of the bog of my despondency like frogs, little geysers of hot spring water spurting out of the mud. This wasn't nearly as bad as the contractions. There was such relief in the act of pushing. There was my own pushing, which was being applauded by the company—everyone was impressed with the speed of things now—but there was also the automatic pushing, the pushing I was designed to do without any prior experience of the act. I felt like a tube of toothpaste, and with every contraction a giant hand would come down and squeeze me in the middle.

"Push into the burning," the nurse said.

And it was true. When I pushed, it burned. That must be skin tearing, I thought. There was less panic in me now. I was approaching joy.

"Okay, his head is almost entirely out. Push! Hold her foot," the nurse told my boyfriend.

I felt lopsided—he had stopped holding my foot. He was entranced by the baby. It pissed me off.

"Hold on to my goddamn foot!"

Then again, "Push!"

"His head is out," someone said. "Don't push."

"I can't!"

"Okay, push."

And then a *swoosh*, an emptying out, like a bucket of swill tipped over, like your own past being hosed out, an erasure, a voiding, and then there was a baby on my belly and he was so big and so familiar I already knew him and seeing him was only confirmation, and he was so gorgeous and so impossible, because how could a human being, which he so clearly was, live in such inhuman conditions, trapped in a wet and claustrophobic sac, although I know that's how we all start out and happily so and that it was this cool and airy room that would be hard for him, a traumatic adjustment, and then he was whisked away to be rubbed from blue to pink and there was the placenta to be born with another voiding *swoosh*, and it was suddenly a pleasant chatty time; I was joking with the doctors, ha ha, ha ha, it was like a cocktail party, and I didn't mind getting stitched up, the pain was a pinprick in comparison, and I could see my boyfriend next to the baby on the other side of the room and I could hear his lusty bawl and then *finally, finally* he was on my chest in a little diaper and a knitted cap and he was clean and so beautiful and exactly the baby I imagined he would be, eight pounds, nine ounces, and I loved the fuzzy apricots of his eyelids and the glassy swirling marbles of his eyes and his fingers like curled rose petals, and I understood at last what it was like to belong to somebody, and I looked at my boyfriend and we exchanged, wordlessly, a prayer in praise of the devastating generosity of the world.

GOD'S RADAR

Michael Redhill

HE WAS BORN COOING, his wet brown eyes reflecting the lights in the ceiling. They laid him on Anne's stomach and he seemed to search above him, a different heavens than the one he was used to. "It's a boy!" I called down the hall, and a small roar went up in the lounge. Back in the room, we traded him back and forth, exhausted and unbelieving.

"Brought in from the cosmos," I said. I thought I saw stars in his eyes.

Two days later, he was gaunt and unhappy. The cry we'd missed in the delivery room filled our hours. It was as if he'd decided to turn back. He wasn't getting food, although he sucked, and his diapers filled with tarry, black feces. The morning of the third day, he was fevered. We brought him to the hospital and they took him away from us and told us he'd need a spinal tap. To rule out meningitis. We sat in the brightly coloured atrium of the Hospital for Sick Children and rocked back and forth, weeping in terror, and promised him, from the terrible distance that separated where we sat and where they punctured him, that if he made it through this, he'd have a free pass until he was eighteen.

———

I'D DOUBTED I'D EVER be a father. Opportunity and inclination seemed to rule against it. I wasn't against becoming a dad: I'd had a good childhood, as childhoods go, and as role models my imperfect parents were as good as or better than most. But as I got into my twenties it began to look like fatherhood wasn't on the agenda. I'd fully taken the road many people start on but most abandon: common sense had given me a miss and I'd become an artist. Poor, selfish, and with only the vaguest of plans, I wasn't fatherhood material. And if it was a burning desire, there was also the question of who I'd become a parent *with*. I'd looked aslant at the ones across various tables and mattresses and asked myself, *Is she the one?* and had never been sure. I met someone in the early nineties I felt pretty good about, but then she informed me in a letter that there'd been a clerical error and she was going to be spending her life with someone else. I despaired a little after that and embarked on a few years' worth of ill-advised adventures with people crazier, angrier, and more despairing than me, and by the end of my twenties, fathering a child was no longer an issue. It seemed settled to me. I also didn't know very many people who were having kids, since I was living in a world of people who were as unsettled as I was. Into this uncertainty, however, stepped someone who wasn't afraid of it. My good luck, her leap of faith. As we got to know each other, a hint of bigger things returned to my life, and that question came back too, but it was rephrased: *Are we the ones?*

THEY HOOKED HIM TO their machines, as if the tubes and wires were the only things that could keep him with us. Two splints of wood and half a paper cup were tricked up over his intravenous to keep him from accidentally pulling it all out; he kept whacking himself on the head with it and screeching in pain. One morning I had to be held back from attacking a nurse who was being too businesslike with him. Maybe I had the right kinds of instincts after all.

We were riven with anxiety and grief, and the waiting was killing us: the cool-headed doctors said it would take three days to get back the tests that would tell us whether he was meningitic or not. In the meantime they were flooding his system with so much antibiotic it could have turned a tonne of yogurt back into milk.

Also, through one of those tubes, they were feeding him. And his colour returned, his fever went down. I remember ghosts of people entering and leaving the room; they moved in the periphery of our single-minded attention—he yet lived. I don't recall if we ate, if we used the bathroom. I know we didn't sleep. Forty-eight hours in, exhausted and nearly insane, we were "encouraged" to take a walk. Our parents were there and Ben was sleeping. We held hands in the elevator as it whispered us back down into the atrium where we had held each other two days earlier.

I REMEMBER ALL OF ANNE'S pregnancy almost better than I do the actual moment of birth. I realized during it that the long gestation of the human animal is designed solely to get the father ready for a lifetime of responsibility. It's no mistake that the moment of impregnation is called *conception*: at first, parenthood is nothing more than an idea. Then time passes and the evidence of what is coming gets more and more obvious, although for the man, whose body does nothing and who goes through no external changes, the thing that grows inside him is not physical. He begins to form an idea out of this conception, and then the idea becomes a plan. I *will* be a father. I remembered my own parents' mistakes and wondered if I would repeat them. I knew even then that I would. Not the same mistakes, but different ones of the same enormity, ones as inevitable.

She puked through the whole pregnancy. It was supposed to be "healthy," but I couldn't help seeing it as a response to an existential problem. Having a child is sowing the seeds of your own obsolescence: birth is the fuse that leads to that other thing. You appear, you replace yourself, you die. I had preferred to see myself as outside the swim of the normal process of things. As a younger man I'd imagined an unmarried life, unfettered, an artist without ties. Now I lay abed in the mornings with my pregnant partner as she groaned for crackers and cantaloupe, and I knew I was forever on God's radar. It was good to be found.

———

THAT HOUR AWAY FROM Benjamin on what we feared was his deathbed was the most surreal hour either of us had ever passed. We had no strength to walk. We made it just outside the front doors of the hospital and sat on a bench on the sidewalk, letting the sun wash over us. "Are you okay?" "I think so. Are you okay?" "I think so. Look."

There was a tree growing out of one of those concrete donuts on the sidewalk. "That's a tree," one of us said, and the other agreed.

Then we began to laugh. We were sick with laughter. I can't explain it now, but to come downstairs from where our newborn was being urged back towards life and seeing a little sapling standing alone on the sidewalk—it was the most sophisticated joke we'd ever been told. We held on to each other and laughed as if we were going to die. I'm quite sure, even now, that had we laughed a second longer, we would have died. They would have found us on the pavement, the tears streaming down our faces, our mouths locked in a rictus of hilarity. Luckily we got a grip on ourselves and went back upstairs.

They were unplugging Ben from the machines. He's going to be fine, they told us. It was nothing. These things happen. They kept him another night to get the full dose of the antibiotic into him, just in case, and then they sent us home. I filmed us taking him into the house, fully ours at last. But I was so out of it that all I have of the momentous homecoming is a full minute of my mother-in-law's bottom moving up the stairs. She had the baby in her arms. But in the film I can hear him. He's cooing.

———

THE LAST MOMENTS BEFORE he arrived, when his head was out and only Anne's last pushes were to come, the awareness washed over me that mere instants separated me from the last moment in my life when I wasn't necessary to the first moment when I was. This thought frightened me, as I imagine it should frighten any sensible person. You can love those who are going to leave you—either because they precede you or because they can leave you if they choose to — and you can love in the dark knowledge of this. Your parents will die, your loved ones may suffer a change of mood and move on. But to begin to love someone you know *you* will leave, because nature must have it so, is a very heavy thing indeed. Here came the boy who would bury me. Whom I would love for the rest of my life, but not for all of his. I was bringing him into future loss. There is nothing more beautiful or dreadful than this.

And then someone seemed to ask me, *Are you sure?* and held him away from me. *Yes,* I said, *I am sure. I'll give my life.*

———

THIS MORNING BENJAMIN, WHO turned nine in September, was making "soup" in the kitchen sink out of leek cuttings, Pringles, chicken bones, hot water, and dish soap. There was oily water all over the counter, soap bubbles on his shirt, and the sickening scent of soggy potato chips wafting everywhere. I wanted to kill him. Then I remembered he has nine more years of carte blanche. He's lucky. Again.

I often wish I could go back to our younger selves, paralyzed with fear in the cold atrium of Sick Kids, and reassure them that their son would be making a hell of a mess in the kitchen in 2007, but we wouldn't have heard; we were inconsolable and unreachable. Love kept us whole those days, nothing else.

Nature has a way of making you forget the terrors it has in store for you, and we had a second son two and half years later. That one, at the age of ten months, plummeted down the escalator at a downtown Loblaws, strapped into the shopping cart, and survived. Not a scratch. Lost the eggs, though. And apart from a couple of hernias and the regular passel of coughs and colds, neither child has been sick a day. I write this with every digit crossed. And I say to whomever is in charge of these things: remember, please, we paid in advance.

ROAD TRIPS

Sandra Martin

MY HUSBAND WAS AT the wheel on our annual trek to Prince Edward Island, while I slouched in the passenger seat, idly tracking ornamental wishing wells on manicured rural lawns. Such are the companionable pursuits of a long-journeyed couple as the kilometres click by, especially now that our children are grown and have found their own travel modes and companions. I no longer referee brawls, nurse babies to sleep, read chapter books aloud, play Name That Tune and I Spy, or try to ignore the heavy metal vibes of Metallica and the vicious lyrics of 50 Cent. My husband and I have reclaimed our interrupted sentences and our solitary thoughts — and most of the time we revel in that.

Or so I was thinking when a modulated female voice on a radio phone-in show distracted me from my wishing-well survey. The topic was doctor shortages and escalating health-care costs, and the caller, a family doctor, was saying how she preferred to treat men rather than women. Their bodies aren't as complicated — apparently a prostate exam is faster, cheaper, and requires less equipment than a Pap smear. Besides, she said, men don't go into labour in the middle of the night and disturb her sleep, or make other patients cranky because they have taken up too much time in her examining room with their teary anguish about delinquent mates and wayward children. Men are easier to service, more cost-effective, and far less emotionally taxing. As a small businesswoman, she needed to take those factors into account.

The harassed family doctor's explanation was perfectly plausible, but it chilled me. I don't blame her for putting efficiency over empathy — at least she was honest about her priorities. How can she have time to listen when she has tests to conduct, paperwork to complete, a living to earn? She's not alone in that. Most of us are too isolated or preoccupied to concentrate on the attenuated details of other people's lives. And that is when I felt sad for what the doctor was missing as she clocked her way through life. But in that moment I also understood why I had agreed to write this essay about birth stories.

We are all born and we all eventually die, but it is only women who grow a fetus and bear children in what is surely the largest physical incident of our lives. And yet that event is rarely represented in visual art or literature or music — especially from the perspective of the mother. Birth stories are fomented in gutwrenching physicality, but the irrepressible desire to tell them comes from an urge to make our experience larger than ourselves and to embed it in a universal maternal continuum. We write our stories to make sense of that first breathtaking moment when our children separate from our bodies and begin to become their own individual selves on a journey that takes them away from us.

ABOUT MY OWN BIRTH, I know little. My parents were married after my father came back from serving as a radar officer for four bloody years on capital ships in the Royal Navy during the Second

World War. Barely ten months after the wedding my older sister was born. If they could have prevented or delayed me they would have, for my father was a doctoral student at McGill, helping to build the first cyclotron in Canada, and my mother was almost crippled with pain because her first pregnancy had aggravated an old back injury. She was Catholic and he was unsophisticated, and so I was set to emerge fifteen months after my sister's arrival.

What to do with the first child while she was in hospital having the new baby was a taxing problem for my mother, as it is for so many of us. There were no grandparents able to help. So one of my father's sisters — childless and fifteen years his senior — agreed to stop over with her husband on their late fall migration from the Niagara Peninsula to PEI and stay with us in the huts, as student housing at McGill University was aptly called.

Every morning, as November turned bleaker and the crowded hut became more claustrophobic, my aunt would turn to my mother and say, "Do you think it will be today, dear?" After a week of question period, my mother begged her doctor to do something and he did: he put her in hospital and induced her. "I'll never do that again," was all my mother would say later about the racking and relentless spasms that preceded my birth. The best part, apparently, was lying alone in her hospital bed afterwards, away from the demands of family and listening to the radio broadcast of the wedding of Princess Elizabeth to the Duke of Edinburgh. In gratitude, she gave me Elizabeth as a middle name.

THE SUMMER I WAS FIVE, my mother took my older sister and me by train from Kingston, where we lived, to PEI, so that we could spend six weeks with my father's widowed mother and a clutch of his older sisters while he gave a training course to navy recruits in Halifax. It was an oddly brave thing for her to do on her own, for her marriage to my father, which crossed the religion bar, had been hotly contested.

I can remember nervously climbing a ladder on the swaying train, opening the curtains on the upper berth, and fearing I would fall into a rabbit hole like Alice, and then waking up the next morning to see rumpled men in raincoats stumbling down the aisle to the bathroom. The forested landscape whizzed by the windows until finally I could feel the train chug into the belly of the ferry for the seaward part of the journey.

My mother, wearing a dress with a cinched waist and a hat on her head, led us decorously up the red-carpeted stairs of the old SS *Abegweit*. I clung to the polished brass railing as I climbed from one step to another until we finally reached the glamorous swirl of the passenger deck, where grown-ups were drinking highballs and eating lobster at tables draped with white linen cloths.

Through the glass windows we had our first glimpse of the red soil and green fields of the island, lying across the sparkling blue waves of the Northumberland Strait. So much happened that summer — the dunes, the tides, the jellyfish, the beginning of an abiding love for my aunts — that it is still the most vivid summer of my life. And that is another kind of birth: the emergence of an overwhelming sense of belonging to a particular place.

BY THE TIME I WAS pregnant, in 1979, childbirth had changed from solitary teeth-gritted pain or anesthetic-induced amnesia into a communal experience complete with prenatal breathing and coaching classes. My husband and I had a birth kit prepared that included pillows, tennis balls, face cloths, a lunch in case he got hungry, soothing music on cassettes, an instruction book, and enough other useless paraphernalia to fill an overnight case.

We were far from extreme in our preparations. A couple we met in Lamaze class actually made a pact that he would refuse to let her have an epidural even if she screamed for drugs. Not me. I was hoping for a natural birth, but I had no desire to be a hero. To tell you the truth, my biggest concern was whether I was capable of being a mother. I knew I could handle the work and the responsibility, but I wasn't sure I could love a baby, with its demands and its interruptions, more than the ancient cat on whom I lavished affection.

All of that existential angst evaporated just before 5:00 a.m. on a Friday morning in late July, three days past my due date. The previous evening my sister and I had finished papering the baby's room—or rather, she had climbed a ladder with paste and paper and I had staggered around offering her praise and the occasional beer.

So these are the contractions I'm supposed to ignore for the next eight hours, I thought, remembering the last lesson in our Lamaze classes. That's when I doubled over from the next tsunami of pain. Ten minutes later I had called the doctor, woken my husband, and kissed the cat goodbye. My husband went out to find the car—one of the delights of urban living is trying to remember where you parked the night before. By now the pains were five minutes apart. In the scramble to get me into the front seat, we forgot the equipment bag, which meant another delay while my husband went back to the house to retrieve it.

"You'd better not be thinking about natural childbirth, because you aren't going to make it," a nurse said to me when I leaned against the wall during a particularly powerful contraction, as she led me down a long corridor to a labour room while my husband searched for a place to stow the car. By the time he found me again, the nurse had examined me and grudgingly admitted I was four centimetres dilated. Twenty minutes later the contractions seemed constant and erratic, but I knew that couldn't be, because I had read the book.

"Do you want something for the pain?" a new nurse asked, poking her head around the door. She came over to examine me and blurted, "I can't find the cervix," as she raced for the doorway.

"Where did it go?" I demanded irrationally.

"Do you want to push?" she asked, turning around as I jack-knifed on the bed.

So that's what the urge to push feels like, I realized, numbly nodding my head as tremors from another earthquake threatened to cleave my body apart.

"Well, don't," she ordered. "I'm calling the doctor."

The doctor must also have had trouble finding his car, because after waiting forty minutes for him to arrive, the nurses woke up a resident. All this time they kept ordering me not to push, as though my splayed and unmedicated body and heaving belly could be cajoled into passivity.

My husband swears that I had snarled, "Forget it, I've had enough. I'm getting out of here," and was yanking one heel out of the stirrup when my doctor finally burst into the delivery room, eyes blazing at the nurses. By now the frustrated baby had started moving backwards up the birth canal and had to be persuaded to come down again. Even so, in less than four chaotic hours from that first twitch before dawn I had a baby nuzzling my chest.

His maleness amazed me. I come from a family of women—three sisters, six aunts—and it simply never occurred to me that I would have a boy. All I wanted was for everybody to go away so that I could explore this strange little creature. But instead he was taken away to have a bath, and I was stashed in a corridor to rest until they could find me a bed in the maternity ward.

The thing about a rapid delivery, aside from the danger of hemorrhaging, is that it leaves you pumped with adrenalin and feeling exhilarated rather than exhausted. I could have climbed mountains, run marathons, swum the Channel. Instead I lay there fretting that the nurses would bring me somebody else's baby and I wouldn't know because I hadn't memorized him yet. We phoned our relatives to pass the time, and then we demanded our son. When the nurse wheeled him in, tightly wrapped like a papoose and lying on his side in a plastic crib, I looked at his scrunched little face and I knew he was mine. He was the other, but he had my forehead and my eyes, and when I finally held him, he fitted in my arms as though he had been pre-moulded to my body shape. I knew I would always know him.

HAVING GROWN UP CROWDED against an older sister, I luxuriated in the solitary hours with my son. He was the focus of my days—wakeful, alert, yet calm—a self-regulating baby who slept at night. Realizing how smug I must have been about my perfect child, who never suffered from colic or earache, makes me cringe retroactively. I can still remember glancing sideways at him in his crib when he was about six months old and realizing with a shock that perhaps he wasn't the most beautiful baby I had ever seen in my life.

I happily obeyed the parenting books that prescribed a three-year wait before trying to conceive a sibling for him. The second time around, I knew pregnancy's payoff—a child who would stretch my emotional tendrils from joy to fear—and I knew who I was—a woman who had been enhanced, disciplined, and energized by motherhood.

Everybody said I must be hoping for a girl, but I refused to think about the sex of the fetus in my rapidly expanding belly.

Over the decades my mother had made it abundantly clear that at least one of her four daughters should have been a male, to compensate for the horrific deaths of her two younger brothers, aged nineteen and twenty-one, in a boating accident before any of us was born. Being superfluous and yet too flimsy to balance the weight of that loss was not a burden I wanted to pass on to my unborn child. Besides, it was a baby I wanted, not a symbol.

As the summer grew steamier and my joints became swollen, I had to soak myself in a warm bath every morning before I could bend my knees or squish my lumpy feet into flip-flops. I had nightmares in which my husband was out of town, the pains racked my body at two-minute intervals, and my son clutched at my skirt while I frantically searched for the car keys. "Metro woman gives birth in back seat of cab while older child watches" was the fantasy headline that invariably woke me in a cold sweat. I could see why women like my mother opted for induction. They could wash the kitchen floor, drop the older children off at the sitter's, and head for the hospital for a scheduled birth.

In fact, my second birth story was mostly the stuff of soft music and rosy videos, with the requisite peaks of dramatic tension. On a muggy Sunday afternoon, once again three days past my due date, I was kneading blue food colouring into playdough at the picnic table in our garden while my son and my husband worked on a wooden jigsaw puzzle, when I felt a gush and realized my waters had broken. They were green, which meant the baby had passed meconium in utero and might be in distress.

And yet everything worked. My doctor was away but his substitute answered the phone, listened to what I was saying, and told me to go to the hospital right away; my sister was at home and offered to take our son to the Superman movie that had just opened; the nurses at the hospital were gracious and helpful — and laughed when I explained why my fingernails were blue. They hooked me up to a monitor, praised the length and depth of my contractions, and showed me how strongly the baby's heartbeat was registering. We'd forgotten to pack a lunch for my husband in the birth kit and so he wandered off to find a sandwich. He was back quickly, but I hadn't missed him because this was all about the baby and me. We were in perfect sync — nobody else mattered — and then there she was, big, lusty, and flashing a crest of flaming red hair.

"If I weighed nine pounds and was trying to push my way through a birth canal, I'd have a bowel movement too," said the nurse.

Where has she come from? I wondered, as I cradled this feisty child, who had been conceived within days of my own mother's harrowing death from breast cancer and who had burst from my body after ninety minutes of labour. Nobody grabbed the baby from me, so I could hold her bloody, amniotic fluid– and meconium-streaked body as she nuzzled and sniffed my sweaty skin. She was female, but she had my husband's body shape and colouring and looked nothing like me at all. Most of all, she had *red hair* — that was the most surprising aspect, because I come from a long line of brunettes and stupidly thought that all my children would look like me. And yet this mysterious amalgam of our recessive genes, this person who has none of our reserve, mordant self-consciousness, or caution, has been the tempestuous dynamic that turned us from a couple with the "perfect only child" into a family.

But it gets better. After an hour or so a nurse came to my room to ask if she could bathe the baby, and promised to bring her back as soon as she was cleaned up. Within minutes of the nurse wheeling the baby, bundled tightly in a pink blanket in her

Plexiglas bassinette, into the hospital room, our almost-four-year-old son arrived with his aunt, both of them full of excitement about the Superman film they had just seen.

"Come and see what we have for you," my husband said, and led him gently towards his little sister. She wasn't of much interest, if truth be told, but he was much taken with the gaily wrapped parcel that was lying beside her.

"Who's that for?" he asked.

"Have a look," I said from my bed. "She brought it with her as a present for you."

And with that he ripped open the parcel to reveal a blue Superman T-shirt with a red cape trailing from the shoulder seams. The ideal gift from his new little sister, so perfect, in fact, that he wore it every day for the next six months. I'd like to say that every day was as blissful as that one, but you wouldn't believe me. Besides, joy has no resonance without the contrast of the sadness, worry, boredom, and frustration that are an inevitable component of parenthood.

We gave our daughter the two family names we had planned to bestow on our first-born, until he turned out to be male, and added a third in memory of my mother — the grandmother she would never know. And when we made the difficult but sensible decision to have no more than two children, I mourned that my daughter would never have a sister. The fact that my beloved son would never have a brother is a lament that occurred to me only years later.

WE ALWAYS TALK ABOUT raising children, but I think we learn at least as much from them as they do from us. My son taught me to work ferociously when he napped and to slow down when we went for a walk as he circled trees, poked with sticks, and splashed in puddles like a dog let off its leash. And he exposed me to maleness—the wrestling, the urge to kick balls, to pick up sticks from the ground that he invariably transformed into impromptu guns and swords, the ability to play games with packs of random boys, to build weapons of mass destruction out of Lego, and the rough physicality of his embraces—the strangleholds that camouflaged the need for a hug.

My daughter taught me spontaneity, exuberance, and passion. Her social interactions were so much more complicated than his. Instead of kicking back a ball or chasing a kite, she and her playmates executed delicate and sometimes vicious social negotiations about who was the chief princess or who got to wear the beaded veil while playing dress-up. She loved Lego too, but not as a building tool. For her, constructions made from the plastic bricks were stage sets for fantasies about love, death, and betrayal.

What we all shared was reading, although they listened in totally different ways. She clung with her head plastered to my armpit, while he roamed the room and pretended to take shots on goal. From the beginning, reading was a weapon—they would both stay in their cribs for afternoon naps if they had a stack of picture books to "read"—a diversion, and a consolation. Once during a play date, when a new friend got homesick and began to cry, my three-year-old son ran out of the room and returned with a tattered copy of *Goodnight Moon* under his arm. Reading was also the way I could cuddle him under one arm while I nursed the baby as the three of us snuggled in my bed. And it was always the ploy I used to calm my tempestuous daughter, although, despite her red hair, she thwarted me with *Anne of Green Gables*. Finally, after lots of cajoling, she allowed me to read the book to her, and then gently wiped the tears streaming down my face when we got to the part where Matthew dies. That was the first but not the last time I have been astonished by my daughter's insouciant capacity for empathy.

There was another ritual we shared. On their birthdays my husband and I would wake them with croissants, juice, and hot chocolate. As they chomped I would sit on their beds and repeat the familiar tale that always began with me saying, "I remember the day you were born..." and ended with a description of how they looked and felt the first time I held them in my arms. Now on their birthdays, instead of breakfast in bed I wake them with an early morning phone call, and they are as likely as not to jump-start my romantic reverie by intoning in melodramatically choked voices, "I remember the day..."

AS THE YEARS PASSED, my children went off to summer camp, holidays with friends, trekking in Europe, and to attend universities that were far enough away from home to establish a distance, but not so remote as to send an irrevocable message. There are stacks of snapshots recording those departures. In one respect they are always the same: I am wearing dark glasses so as not to embarrass them, or me, with my welling eyes, and I am invariably clutching one of them by the arm or the shoulder. They have long since marked their independence when it comes to holidays, and mostly that is fine with me as I remind myself of the mantra my father often chanted about family visits: so nice to have them come, so nice to see them go.

But then my father died suddenly of a stroke. My husband and I went to PEI as usual that summer. Walking by the sea, knowing how much of my father I had inherited in my love of the spray and roar of the waves, I was convulsed with sadness and loss. I was inconsolable. Then my grown children, who had never really shared my passion for the Island, arrived in a rented car to bunk in with us for a week, using up their precious vacation time to ease me through my grief. And I realized, as we swam, played cards, ate lobster, drank wine, read books, and walked forever at low tide, that without them my journey would have been soulless.

ANIMALIA

Pauline Holdstock

IT'S DARK. THE BED is cold. I'm cold. The shivering began a while ago. It's turned to a convulsive shuddering and I can't keep still. The single blanket is not nearly enough. Somewhere a baby has begun to cry. It's down the hall somewhere, quite far. The voice of an infant lost, abandoned. The clear vowels of want and need, the language of distress itself. Someone, please. I speak this language. I speak it. This baby is all alone, unattended. Please. I want it to stop. Instead it's getting louder. The voice clambers over the wreckage of its wretchedness and rises to get a hold on solid rage and proclaim its desperation. I speak this language. I know how to answer it. But it's moving farther away and there's nothing I can do.

Traces of unhappiness escape into a distant hallway, the clamorous, craving child now sorely affronted. I need to get up. There is nothing at hand to staunch the blood. Please. This is a hospital. They are surely not hurting him. Please. Someone. The tone changes again, is less angry, but still this child is not getting what he wants. Bring him back. He is mine. I know I have been listening to my own child. I can give him everything he needs, his birthright above all else. His place is here beside me. We are each other's warmth and life.

And of course they do bring him back. They took him away "to clean him up." I imagine him parked in a brightly lit 2:00 a.m. hallway while some hair-raising hospital emergency was satisfactorily resolved. Though his was an emergency. In his two-hour-old world a desperate emergency. Life and death.

I imagine him when his turn came. Soap-smelling hands lift him from his parking spot, lay him in the baby-rest on the steel table and unwrap him the way I unwrap fish on the kitchen counter. And there the resemblance ends, because this fish is warm and pink with out-flung limbs — starfish! — working the air with a red, open mouth and equipped with a tight, bawling barrel of sound for a chest.

The hands pick him up and dunk him quickly in the plastic bath, where the cooling water feels like loss itself. The hands scrub away his past life, rub off the very essence of himself, removing the only smell he knows. They lift again, pat, wrap, trap what remains of his heat.

"But this child is a vocalist!" says the voice belonging to the hands that draw back the single blanket and lay the screamer beside me in the bed.

"Do you need any help?"

I shake my head. I'm remembering the words of a London nurse, spoken to my mother at the birth of her first child and often repeated for the pleasure of all they stand for. Fretful because the newborn would not latch on when first put to the breast, my mother had called the nurse and confessed with a good deal of anxiety that she didn't know what to do. The nurse, who was big in all directions and black and very, very kind, had smiled.

"Never worry, love," she said, and patted her softly on the arm. "You'll think of something…"

My breasts are shot through with a delicious current of energy. They are full to bursting and not just warm. They are hot, could start an engine on a Saskatchewan morning in January. My baby's mouth is clamped on hard and he's drowning in the sudden supply, but he's not crying.

Ah, but this bed is no cold rectangle of Saskatchewan drive-way. This bed is Christmas under a goose-down duvet. It's a July night with a full moon and no mosquitoes. It's a soft pink beach in the Caribbean. It's a fragrant loaf fresh from the oven, and we are inside it, breathing.

THE BIRTH, MY THIRD, had been easy—as births go—uncompli-cated, devoid of trauma or surprise. Best of all, I had been handed my child immediately, had tucked him down beside me and put him to the breast. We had both fallen asleep, rocked by the rise and fall of our breath, blanketed in the warmth of our bodies. The comfort we both felt—how do I know "both"? Trust me—was the deep and untroubled peace of absolute security. I think I was aware even then of its precious nature. It was a satiety derived from lack. No hunger, no pain. No worries. Pretty much a definition of heaven. A kind of morphic bliss without the mor-phine. Feather pillows all around. Swansdown.

IT'S BECOME COMMONPLACE TO say that we forget the pain of childbirth. Every mother can vouch for the truth of the state-ment. The obliteration of the pain is a kind of built-in insur-ance against extinction. But if we know this with our rational minds, why can't we cheat the mechanism, step aside, as it were, and nail the experience in language? It isn't possible. The birth experience happens—like sex, or most likely, death—in a place beyond words. It takes the mother back to the essence of primal being, where existence is experienced raw, is lived wholly, with no intermediary of language or social context. In the white-hot core of the experience, mind and body are fused absolutely. The brain attends only to the business of the body. When there is no mind to do the minding, no self to say *this hurts*, there is only the pain itself. The mother *is* the pain.

At the birth of my second child a little piece of my mind did detach. As a consequence, I realized that I was *being* what was happening, and for a few moments I had words to approximate the experience. I was a kind of airy hourglass cage of white wicker, three-dimensional and hollow, tensile, elastic. The image is not what I recall now, nor even what I "saw" at the time. It is what I *was*, and the experience was unaccompanied by words of any kind. At intervals my being—this flexible cagey construction—turned impossibly outwards on itself. The closest I can come to describing in words what was happening is to say, Imagine a Moebius strip, that three-dimensional model of infinity. Now imagine an hourglass with the same ability to turn itself inside out—for want of a better term, because, like the Moebius strip, this shape has no inside, no outside.

All right, I've gone completely mad—but I hope I've made my point. I can only very hazily approximate the experience, and it has nothing whatever to do with pain. In this wordless place there is no expressing the pain. You *are* the pain, so there is no more you to register it. What I have since pieced together is that my experience of being the wicker cage—which it doesn't take much to decode as the pelvis—occurred at one of the most painful moments of the birth: the point of transition, where full dilation of the cervix is reached. So if you were to interrogate me on the pain of that moment, I wouldn't have much to tell you. I was otherwise occupied. *I*, in fact, wasn't there.

I HAVE A PICTURE OF my firstborn, a few hours old. Her sweet face is horribly reddened and marked. In the midst of all the pushing and grunting I was doing, I was told by a voice—another disembodied voice—that the doctor was going to use lower forceps. I would rather have gone on pushing but the voice told me the forceps were necessary and would be okay. Somehow *lower* became equated with *lesser*. So, okay. I don't know how I missed the point, in all the prenatal education I absorbed, that using lower forceps means reaching into the birth canal to get hold of the baby's head with a pair of tongs like the ones I use on the barbecue.

I'd wanted a natural birth. I'd wanted a midwife, but they were illegal in B.C. I'd wanted to stay at home, but that was not an option, and I wasn't brave enough to go it alone like my Navajo friend who went into the B.C. bush with her husband to deliver her third child. I would have liked to be in a birthing home that would afford privacy, dignity, time, plus assistance if things went pear-shaped. But such places existed only in the minds of a few enlightened visionaries. All right then, if it had to be a hospital, I made it clear that I did not want on any account to give birth on my back, a position that induced intense pain even without contractions. But my endless exhortations and pleas were like the cries of Brer Rabbit. Please don't throw me in the briar patch. I ended up, of course, in a sterile delivery room, supine. I cannot remember the pains of the contractions, not one. But I can remember the severe and nauseating pain of that position. I can feel it now.

They did at least give me my daughter straightaway. The experience of pain, even the pain of an intern's clumsy tailoring, was already melting, dissolving. Nothing was as vital as this warm, quick little being in my arms. A few hours later, at peace in the warm bed, gazing in that besotted maternal manner I seem to have mastered in a heartbeat, I inhaled deeply, catching the clean, dry scent of vernix — or the last traces of it. Vernix is the waxy covering that protects the fetus. It's the substance the hospital staff work so conscientiously to remove. It smells a little like beeswax — wholesome, slightly sweet — but is really like no other substance you'll ever encounter. Overcome, I fought the desire to bend my face to my newborn and taste. I tried to think of other things. I wish I had licked. I know we would have both enjoyed it.

———

THE URGE TO LICK was certain evidence of the animal nature we've smothered under layers of civilization. Everything about the birth experience is veined and marbled with that forgotten nature. I think it's the reason the pregnant woman and the young mother slip into an altered state — at least I did — behaving alternately like a somnolent dairy cow and an enraged tigress. (And it never completely disappears. The latter surfaced recently in a bank when I was blocked from putting money in my son's account. Since he was in difficulty in a foreign country and in need of a doctor, the enraged tigress woke up and sprang from nowhere. She got what she wanted. Indeed, she probably could have robbed the place. The offspring, by the way, was twenty-five...) And those two opposing states, the pacific and the ferocious, might single-handedly account for the nature of Kali Ma, the Hindu deity who is both creator and destroyer. Both womb and tomb, she devours her children — a practice unconscionable to mere humans (and likely the reason I didn't dare taste the vernix, in case a nurse happened by and assumed the worst). But there is another, more potent explanation.

At the moment of delivery, while my child was still slippery from the passage, I had seen my own blood on her head. The symbolism was blatant and the immensity of what I had just done came home to me. I had given life, and with it, death. Indeed, a terrible power—one we do well to relegate to a nonhuman being lest we go mad. The urge to apologize was as powerful as the urge to push. The human and the animal. I didn't talk about the appalling truth. As we do with our own mortality, I kept it out of sight, in a locked room. A month or two later, an aged neighbour voiced it. When, all maternal pride and beaming, I showed her my sleeping child, she eschewed the platitudes. Instead she laid her papery palm on the baby's head.

"There," she said. "If you knew, if you only knew."

The same human consciousness that makes us aware of mortality also has us striving to outwit it, to make backup copies against the inevitable. Join that mechanism with sheer animal impulse and you have a potent combination, one that can easily make a full-fledged family in no time.

That powerful instinct has permeated, I see now, all my fiction. It's never far away.

To perform the stunt so dangerously close to the edge was exhilaration of a kind of which she would never tire.
To see life turn at the last, the first moment and clutch at the wind-blown grass with star-shaped hands, feet perfect like little fish flying above the dark and eyes amazed and looking. For her. This was living.

THREE YEARS HAVE PASSED since my little son had his chilly bath along the hospital hallway. I am taking him on an outing with his grandmother, visiting from England, and his new baby sister. We have arrived at the aquarium to view the sea lions, reputed to enjoy performing for visitors—which may well be true, for that is the time they are fed dripping bucketfuls of herring. Whether they enjoy the rest of their days and nights in captivity is a moot point.

We are pleased with ourselves for having organized our party to be arriving in good time for the first performance. Tracking lost socks, diaper bag, car keys, juice boxes, Ninja Turtles, and the two tiny pet caterpillars (rolled from tiny scraps of playdough) that must accompany us everywhere has been no mean feat when the search team is so easily distractible. Nevertheless, here we are at the green-painted ticket booth a full five minutes before the show. Naturally we are dismayed and hugely disappointed when we are told that today there will be no first performance. We put on our own show—Customer Dissatisfaction, featuring indignant patrons practised in complaints. We lend weight to the exhibition with suppressed but audible mutterings and, from one of the party, expressive battering of the ticket office with the toe. The attendant is impressed and relents.

"Well, you can go in anyway," she says. "I won't charge you. But there'll be no show. One of the females has just given birth."

My mother and I exchange glances, raise eyebrows. We try not to look too delighted at the prospect of an exhibition that promises to outclass any tourist act. The privilege!

We make our way around and up through the passage that leads to the viewing area around the open pool. A waist-high wall separates the tiered seating from the almost oval tank. The tank, circumscribed by a narrow deck, is unnaturally blue, like a swimming pool. At the blunt end is a wider deck with four doors giving on to it, closed for now, and a high fence behind. Two men have taken up positions on a narrow catwalk that projects from the wider deck into the middle of the pool. A lifeguard's chair stands ready at one side with its various poles and props beside it, several balls, a series of hoops.

We are the first visitors of the day, the only spectators, for as we shall see when we leave, there is now a chalked notice of cancellation outside the entrance. We stand at the wall. My mother holds the baby while I lift my son to see. And there, there she is, the mother, between the two men on the catwalk. The men move apart briefly and we get a good view. There is no analogy for the blackness or the glossy liquidity of this animal. She is beautiful. If night were made water... The loosely connected trio shuffle and slide down the catwalk to the wider deck, and the men step aside. There! We spot it. The pup! She keeps it close to her belly. How this tiny replica blends with her. One of the men picks up the end of a coiled hose and turns it on. Ah, but this now is a show, for look at her! She bares her throat and belly to the stream of cool water. She has the pup directly in front of her and her upper body rears and weaves above it in maternal ecstasy. She dips down to the newborn, sweeps her face above it, and then is up again, stretching her neck in what we take to be pleasure and pride.

The men too are doing their own quirky dance. When she turns they turn. Now she is sweeping her belly and neck over the pup. She is bending over it, making motions with her head, sweeping, stroking. Is she licking? Do sea lions lick? But the men are in the way. It is hard to see. They have poles now. Something changes. The pup is suddenly separated from the mother. The men move swiftly. It's not poles but brooms they have, and one man is fending off the mother while the other is pushing the pup over the deck towards the doors, and in a flash it is done. The pup has been shovelled offstage, as it were, and is behind one of the closed doors. The mother is beside herself with distraction. She plunges along the deck. There is no more fending her off. The second man ducks through one of the other doors to safety. The mother screams in her hoarse voice for the pup. She lunges at the place where it disappeared. She rises up and flings herself vertically at the door. Again and again she hurls herself against it. Her shining body slams into the wood, and she does not stop calling in her harsh, broken voice.

It is not what we have come to see—not what we would ever want to see. My mother has tears in her eyes. We can barely speak to each other as we turn away, unable to watch this public performance. I'm shaking as I go back to the ticket office, don't quite know what to say except it is not right. I hear myself repeating again and again: *It is not right.*

We obtain, of course, repeated assurances. It is the way things are done. The pup has to be removed from the mother. It has to be cleaned up. Checked out. She might harm it if they stay together. And they'll be needing the pool for the 11:30 performance.

And something else. But my mother and I are not listening. Nor are we speaking. We are moving away, trying to distance ourselves from the shame of the spectacle, every cell in our bodies electric with need, remembering.

GOBSMACKED

Martin Levin

GOBSMACKED. I THINK THAT'S THE word I want. I thought about bushwhacked. Too cowboyish. *Coup de foudre* (too pretentious, too romantic). Thunderstruck (too elemental). No, gobsmacked is exactly what I want.

It's a combination of *gob*, northern Brit colloquial for mouth, and *smacked*, which means "utterly astonished, astounded." It's much stronger than just being surprised; it's used for something that leaves you speechless or otherwise stops you dead in your tracks. It suggests that something is as surprising as being suddenly hit in the face.

It's a new word in common parlance, but then this was a new creature I was responding to, and an entirely new experience. Which I suppose I ought to explain.

What gobsmacked me was the birth of my first child, for which I was prepared only notionally. Oh, sure, being a decent enough husband *moyen sensual* and a family-oriented Jewish boy, I was visibly onside with pretty much all my then-wife's prenatal decisions: get pregnant, stop smoking and drinking, perform all

appropriate prenatal rites such as birth classes and Lamaze training, prepare for natural childbirth, help with breathing exercises,
be there during delivery for encouragement and frottage (as
opposed to the old ritual of drinking and smoking—but then,
I had given those up, hadn't I?—in the Anxious Fathers' Waiting
Room), generally be loving and supportive, and never, never
display the slightest doubt that fatherhood—which inevitably
involves the appearance of a child—is exactly what you've been
craving ever since you became an adult (which for many of us is
perpetually *mañana*).

But let's back up a little. At this point, K. and I had been
married for five years—and were to survive in some variant of
coupledom for eleven more years and four more births. Among
the prods I was given towards full adulthood—or, as I like to call
it, creeping post-adolescence—was K.'s burning desire to produce heirs and assigns, which she persisted in calling children or,
more alarmingly, babies. In short, she craved kids. Lots of kids.
K. was born with her biological clock in full tick.

I, on the other hand, gave the matter little thought other than
the lightly held idea that it was incumbent on me to be obliging,
and that a bairn or two might be a nice... what? Addition?
Playmate? Connubial bribe? Perhaps a partial discharge of my
obligation to help replenish the frequently massacred Jewish
tribe? Also, if K. wanted kids, could I, who purportedly loved
her—who actually did love her—refuse her that contemplated
bliss?

No, I could not. But I could deploy what marital wits I might
muster to defer gratification. Hers, not mine. This strategy
involved the inevitable hippie-era European sojourn—nine
months (nudge, nudge) of the Grand Tour in a minor key—and
four years in grad school, much of it spent in bootless fretting

about thesis topics or playing pickup basketball, and wherein responsibility resided chiefly in following the literary fortunes of Mark Twain, Jane Austen, Erasmus, and Samuel Richardson.

Finally, after much negotiation, the occasional tear, some friendly conversation about what it meant to be an adult, the persistent urgings of family members, and a few false starts, there arrived gravidity (which has, I hasten to add, little to do with gravity, a wont of which I was said to suffer). But look, I offered to imaginary inquisitors in defence of my half-decade of resistance, I can recite gobs of Yeats, engage fully in Richardson's two-thousand-page-plus novel *Clarissa*, and even participate in reasonably sophisticated discussion of Plato's *Symposium*. Could a non-adult do that? I asked. Could he? Eh? Huh?

So the evitable became inevitable. But even while K. was preggers, the prospect of a child was somehow unreal. Or unfathomable. The reality consisted of a new lump in a previously svelte belly, the appearance of maternity clothes (I still remember one little number with a Paul Klee design), and plans for the reconfiguration of our apartment. I did not fantasize about watching a daughter dance *Giselle* or a son play ball for the Montreal Expos, nor did I worry about birth defects, though I did wish for K. a delivery that was short and relatively painless. As for the distant prospect of grandfatherhood, which one of my newly childed friends immediately began to mention—heaven forfend! I was, at most, engaged to be engaged, still a father in notion, not essence.

I know, I know, this is commonly thought to be standard among men...er, boys. I am the eldest of four brothers and, in retrospect, had little interest in my new siblings except to consider how their arrival and apparently long-term presence might inconvenience me, or wreck my stuff. In the latter respect they were not bad, although my cherished electric football game, with its tiny red and yellow men vibrating downfield on strips of plastic, did come a cropper. Until they reached an age of modest sentience, when they could be played with, bribed, amused, even — forgive me! — modestly bullied, they were largely a distraction.

Indeed, watching my own sons — to jump ahead a little — only confirmed what I began to suspect was the near universality of this trait, at least among heterosexual North American males of genus Baby Boomer. When one of K.'s friends would show up with the latest addition to her numerous brood, my daughters were willing, even eager to check it out, maybe even coo a little. My sons, though, were — let us be frank — indifferent at best. "Look," K. would say, "here's B. with her new little boy." From my own boys, barely even a polite glance, a distracted nod, before they returned to whatever roughhousing they were enthusiastically engaged in.

So why, aside from metrosexuals (a category of male that, I often think, contains no members) and men cowed into feigned sensitivity, are we so blasé about other people's children? As so often these days, we may turn to Darwin and his followers for enlightenment. By now we all know the theory of the selfish gene as promulgated some thirty years ago by British scientist Richard Dawkins (now more famous as a jeering promulgator of atheism). The theory, in its most reductionist version, states that we humans, in common with all other animals and, indeed, all other living things, are merely conduits for replication, genetic copying machines. (If so, I wish my parents had punched the Enlarge button.) Thus we are not highly tolerant of those whose genes may be competitive with our own.

In *The Selfish Gene*, Dawkins cites American evolutionary biologist R. L. Trivers, who in 1972 advanced the concept of parental investment (P. I.) in a book of that title. He was talking about a mother's investment of care in a child, otherwise known as altruism, but his strictures can be equally well applied to fathers.

Now, altruism is a spongy notion: biological altruism—in which an individual organism acts against its own apparent reproductive interests—is distinguished by sociobiologists from behavioural altruism, which seems to be a matter of deciding to act against one's apparent interests. For the biologist, for whom genetics is all, it is the consequences of an action, and not the intentions, for an individual's reproductive fitness that determine whether any behaviour counts as altruistic.

Those skeptical about such a view may be directed to the animal world, in which "nature, red in tooth and claw" (from Tennyson's "In Memoriam," a long poem said to have provided the widowed Queen Victoria great comfort) might be interpreted as "my genes are more important than yours." Consider nature's big, fierce predators, ecologically sustainable only in limited numbers. One way to limit their numbers is low birth rates. Another is for males—and sometimes females—to kill the offspring of rivals. This is true of bears, crocodiles, and Cape hunting dogs, among others. It is even sometimes true of chimpanzees. So why not humans? Think of Goya's magnificent and terrifying painting *Saturn Devouring One of His Children*, and you'll get the picture. Good thing we have mothers to protect us. Well, good thing for people not born to Joan Crawford or Britney Spears.

So there's a biological side to this indifference, sometimes shading into hostility. But there may be a practical one as well, I have learned. That's the old motivator: fear. To be sure, there's our much-discussed Peter Pannish fear of commitment, fear of giving up parts of our lives deemed essential (just how very many parts is not easily foreseeable), fear of responsibility, and all the other fears we men have been charged with. Much of that may be true, but it's also mostly a matter for sociology texts and newspaper columnists.

More profoundly, there's fear of failure, which comes in so many different shades. Being a father schooled by teaching and example to care for your progeny means that their health, their development, their safety, their education, their very lives are dependent upon you. And, deep in your heart, you know how unfit you are for such a charge.

For such a schooled father, a child entails a lifetime of worry, of fretting, of alarm, most of it amounting to naught—except, perhaps, for removing one more obstacle between you and your first coronary. But, too often (that would be once), something truly frightening does happen, and if you're unlucky, or just inattentive, it's a world-exploding cataclysm.

From almost, but not quite, the moment of birth—not, at least in my case, the moment of conception or of annunciation— the mind is startlingly alive with this theatre of disaster and its horrific possibilities. You watch for signs of mental deficiency and other deformations, for terrible illnesses of which you've never heard, information about which is easily available on the Internet. You read a story such as Lorrie Moore's brilliant "People Like That Are the Only People Here," and the phrase *peed onk* (pediatric oncology) is suddenly a haunting part of your lexicon. Though my children are all adults now, I will refrain from specific examples, owing to the vestigial and primitive fear (the über-rationalist Dawkins would doubtless jeer) that to imagine a catastrophe is to court it, that agents of chaos lurk everywhere and are privy to our darkest fears, which they are only too eager to exploit. I'm sure you can, as they say, relate.

And there's plenty of ammunition for worry.

Think of poor Robert Latimer, the ill-starred Saskatchewan farmer who spent seven years in jail for euthanizing his twelve-year-old daughter, who was crippled in every way imaginable with cerebral palsy and facing a short lifetime of constant pain. Is that what he bargained for? Is that what any of us bargains for? Think too of all those disaster films—comets crashing into earth, burning skyscrapers, exploding volcanoes, overturned ships—especially overturned ships thought to be unsinkable. All of this might be thought of as what T. S. Eliot called an "objective correlative," a set of events or situations that are an objective form of a particular emotion meant to be evoked. Eliot used the term to apply to art, but I find it works in life as well.

Perhaps, though, we might better call it a "disastrous correlative," for the fear that evil may well befall this infant placed in your care by God, or by chance, in the form of genetics. It hardly matters which, since God or chance has convinced you instantly that this is a life you must protect even at the risk of your own.

Though you are rejoicing in the birth and engaged in local fretting—by which I mean the stuff about names and clothing and rituals and sharing—some part of you is aware that, in Nabokov's memorable image from his memoir *Speak, Memory*, the cradle is poised at the edge of an abyss, life but a brief and (you hope) radiant sliver between two eternal darknesses.

But I am sure such dire thoughts did not occur to me in that first gobsmacked moment, when, to my enduring astonishment, I was occupied with falling instantly and forever in love with that tiny, mewling, slightly jaundiced baby, his hair slick and plastered to his scalp with some internal jelly, his lifetime of demands just beginning. His mother already understood that. I never saw her looking more beautiful, more radiant. Readier. Riper. And watching her breastfeeding, something to which I had never given a moment's consideration (the feeding, not the breasts), made me both stupidly happy and surprisingly envious. I think that's because the raw intimacy of that connection was not then available to me.

As I write this I'm watching an episode (ever the multitasker) of the ... *remarkable* is too weak a word, let's call it astonishing BBC TV documentary series *Planet Earth*. This episode is on the world of ice, and I'm watching comically bulky but also inexpressably poignant male emperor penguins, with their overwintering devotion to their unhatched young, a single egg nestled in a sheltering fold above their feet. And this for an entire Antarctic winter: motionless, foodless, uncomplaining.

Yes, I know that this apparent devotion, this altruism, is biologically determined, a survival strategy worked out over millennia in the most unaccommodating environment. But so is mine, even if modified by culture. And then, seeing my first-born son, I really didn't give a damn.

That was at 3:19 a.m., October 31, 1973, at Winnipeg General Hospital, which I left more changed, and forever changed, than I could possibly have bargained for and in ways I could not possibly have understood. And all it took was a few moments, the effects of which would radiate throughout my life, and through the arrival of my other children. (But for them I was not quite so unprepared.) It was Halloween and, in another case of objective correlative (what would I have done without you, Old Possum?), life's tricks and life's treats were all implicit in those first few minutes. It was and is, in a smallish way, my own Big Bang.

BLOOD

Lisa Moore

RECENTLY I ATTENDED PRENATAL CLASSES with Mary, a close friend of mine who had asked me to be her birth coach. We were one of the few same-sex birth partners in the class. The nurse who gave the classes always made sure there was a space in the circle of chairs in case any of the dads felt like they needed air. During the fifth class the nurse talked about blood.

There will be blood.

Don't worry about the blood.

Bleeding. Blood. Blood. Blood.

There was no hope of getting to the door, I realized. I slid out of my chair onto the floor, out cold. The nurse sent all the other birth partners out of the room and made me put my head between my knees. I could not stand. I threw up twice. Mary, nine months pregnant now, found a wheelchair and wheeled me to Emergency as fast as she could. Another nurse checked my vitals, took some of my blood. When she came at me with the tiny needle I clamped my hand over my eyes.

"Is this your birth coach?" she asked Mary.

"She was," Mary said.

MY HUSBAND AND I VIDEOTAPED the birth of our daughter. Fast-forward nine years, and we are having a son. A boy like Steve, I think: kind and calm and super-intelligent and handsome, a boy. A boy!

"You're a VBAC," the nurse says — vaginal birth after Caesarean.

"Pretty brave," she says.

"Brave," I say. "Why? What can possibly go wrong?"

"Plenty," she says. I sit up on one elbow.

I had been at home washing dishes when my water broke. The baby wasn't due for a month, but I knew from the ultrasounds that he was already a little more than seven pounds.

I hadn't experienced labour with my first daughter. I had nearly died during my first birth. But this time I was ready. My son was going to be early, but I was completely ready.

Except I could find only one dry sock. The other sock was still in the dryer, tumbling around by itself. There was a screech of tires outside the house. My sister-in-law wrenched open the front door. It slammed against the wall, knocking down a picture.

"Let's go," Wanda said. "Come on, come on. Move."

"There's no rush," I said. I was serene. I loved being serene. And the contractions were mild. They were kind of beautiful. I sat down to wait for the sock to dry.

Wanda paced the kitchen, jiggling her keys. Then she sat down too. We were both looking at the floor, listening to the sock turn over in the dryer. Then she leapt out of her chair.

"Forget the sock," she yelled. "Forget the goddamn sock."

I had to wear one wet sock and one dry sock to the hospital.

But I was still serene.

I'd had a feast the night before. My friend Medina had thrown a dinner party. I watched her cut an orange in half and squeeze each half between her fists, the juice dripping through her fingers into a pot of shredded beets bubbling on the stove. The colour of those beets, the orange peel. I could taste the colour. Outside her kitchen window Quidi Vidi Lake glittered like a disco ball. She was serving rabbit, and I was ravenous. It was a hunger like I'd never felt before, and I ate and ate and ate.

The next day, washing the dishes, I felt a reverberating *boom* inside me, a big brass gong echoing through a forbidden city. I knew it was the rabbit. It had tasted so wild and full of forest and autumn wet and momentum, all the dark tunnels it had bounded through, and I couldn't get enough of it.

The nurse was reading a magazine. They had turned the lights down low to create mood. I had the CD player and I was listening to Keith Jarrett. Steve was teaching a night class and when he arrived he'd have the video camera. There was a shower if I decided I wanted one. The contractions were still far apart, but they were definitely manageable. What had everyone been complaining about? Clearly I had a deep pain threshhold, I thought. Some women do; some women don't.

But the word *brave* had a sinister ring.

Me: "What can possibly go wrong?"

The nurse: "Well, for instance, your scar from the previous birth could split open during a contraction and you could bleed internally, to death."

"That doesn't happen," I said. The contractions were actually not that beautiful. They were starting to really, really hurt. I hadn't read the birthing literature. Once again, I'd planned to read it in the last month. And once again, there was no last month.

"Sure it does," she said. She turned a page. "Happens all the time."

The previous birth: I'm pregnant with my daughter, and we're renting a giant house on Victoria Street in downtown St. John's. A house that was dirt cheap because it should have been condemned. Four monstrous storeys, empty room after empty room, high ceilings, cobwebs on the chandeliers, the cold blowing through all of the cracks. Sometimes you could see your breath. Steve was writing his master's thesis and teaching at the university. I worked at a feminist magazine in the morning and waitressed in the afternoon. Tips are pretty good when the waitress is visibly pregnant. People shell out fast. They get up and get their own coffee.

I had to walk down Long's Hill to get from the feminist magazine job to the waitressing job. I had a month and a half to go, and I was in a great deal of pain. My legs were swelling, the corrugated mark of my socks imprinted on my calves; the elastic bands of my underwear left red welts. My wedding ring was stuck and my finger was like a sausage. I had to rest at each telephone pole on the way down the hill. Everything hurt. There was a tearing at my ribs, just as if they had been broken. I cried, leaning on the telephone poles. They seemed so far apart from each other.

I went to the emergency ward one night when I could no longer stand the pain. I wanted to see if I could take an Aspirin. I'd found that I couldn't urinate. I was desperate to pee, but I just couldn't. At the hospital they did a quick check and sent me home.

"Probably just stomach flu," the intern said.

At one in the morning that same night I was climbing in and out of the claw-footed tub. The giant flowers on the old-fashioned wallpaper seemed to be throbbing. Steve was trying to hold me, but I couldn't stay still. I couldn't really move either. I was trying to squirm away from the pain. Steve would sit and try to type his thesis, and get up and try to hold me, and sit again. We were both twenty-six years old.

I said that I wanted to go back to the hospital. If I can't take Aspirin, there must be something else.

Steve said, "Bring your toothbrush."

"Why?"

"I think this is it."

"This is not it," I said. "There's a month and a half to go. This cannot be it."

"I think this is it," he said. They admitted me at once, and when I had settled in the hospital room I took out my contact lenses. This was a problem, because I couldn't see, and I wanted to communicate effectively. Somewhere I had picked up, maybe at the feminist magazine, that effective communication would be a good thing in this kind of situation. Birth plan, bedside manner, interfacing with the institution, owning your birth experience, and all that. But I couldn't talk to people if I couldn't see them. There were several bodies in white lab coats standing around my bed, and I couldn't read their expressions. They were getting ready to inject me with something for the pain.

"Excuse me," I said. "I wonder if you could just wait a minute and let me put in my contact lenses? Also, will that stuff you're giving me affect the baby?"

The doctor said to Steve, "Can I see you outside?" They trooped out.

The needle jabbed; pain disappeared. It was gone. It had been there, killing me, and then it was gone and I was floating, utterly painless, euphoric even. *How interesting is pain*, I had a chance to think. *To come and go as it pleases.*

Then Steve was back. He knelt by the bed and took my hand. He said, "Lisa, this doctor says he doesn't like your personality. He has asked you to shut up. Apparently you might die, and they are doing an emergency surgery. They can't waste a second. The thing is, this guy is about to cut you open with a knife, and so I think maybe we should try to stay on his good side."

The doctor had communicated pretty effectively. I shut up.

Toxemia. They don't really know what it is. The baby somehow poisons the mother. The doctor met my mother at the door to my hospital room. They had known each other since childhood.

"We can save the baby," he said. "I don't know if we can save your daughter."

Am I angry with the doctor? Have I, in the seventeen years that followed, found myself now and then standing in front of the bathroom mirror, toothbrush in hand, carrying on a whole conversation with him through gritted teeth? You don't like my personality? You bully, you great ugly thug of a man, you turd, you sexist, pompous, etc. etc.

In his defence, it was an emergency. He had been delivering babies for hours and hours without rest. There had been more than one close call that night. In his defence, I was dying. In his defence, Hello! I'm alive. And my daughter is too.

Immediately after the operation my face swoll up like a pumpkin.

Swoll, I think, is the right word. I was unrecognizable. The night nurse assigned to me came back the next night and did not know who I was. She had to check the chart.

My platelets were down. Way down. Apparently platelets are a big deal. I dragged myself out of whatever drugged underworld I was living in to pump breast milk. My milk was contaminated by the drugs I was taking, but I had to pump if I wanted to breastfeed later. The suction on that industrial pump—it was a monster. The engine was loud, like the engine of a tractor. I flicked the switch and it chugged into action and the milk hit the side of the little bottle and I bonded with the machine.

"Look, honey," I said to Steve, holding up my two ounces. "Look how much I got!"

My poor husband. His wife transformed, overnight, into a puff pastry. She is leaking and swollen and weeping and still not really out of the woods.

There is a picture of Steve with Eva. Most of her, from the top of her head to the tips of her toes, fits into his big hand. Four pounds, five ounces. Steve was not afraid for her the way I was. He had already had one beautiful daughter and knew how to change a diaper and all the other things you have to know. He believed that Eva and I were both going to be fine, even as I was being wheeled into the operating room. He was excited in his flowery paper cap and face mask. Believing we were going to be okay was his job. Somebody had to do it.

They gave me an epidural.

"We're not operating on your toes," the anesthetist said, when I realized, with terror, that I could still wiggle them.

They were about to cut me open.

Here's what it feels like: you feel the drag of the knife; you feel the numb flesh (your flesh) giving way to that knife.

Steve believes everything will be okay, but he's breaking every single bone in my hand.

Slice, slice, slice, goes the little knife.

And then, there she is! There she is, my God, there she is. There she is. There she is. There she is. What are we in the presence of here? What has happened? She's here. She's here. This is really — what is this? This is pure and untouched and so new. The newness. This is such blazing love. God, Steve, look what we did. Look!

This is the biggest thing I've ever felt. Then I'm out cold.

Eva's birth was scary and full of drugs that left a taste in the back of my mouth and knocked me into sleep so black and cloying, smothering, and absolutely void of sensory detail that I imagine I know what it feels like to be dead.

BUT JUST BECAUSE YOU have toxemia once doesn't mean you'll get it again, and here I was in labour, almost ten years later, with my son. And here is the most honest thing I can say about the pain of labour: I was unequal to it. There was more of it than me. Is childbirth beautiful? Yes, it is. Would I do it again? No.

Stamina is an interesting word.

How orderly it all is, the contractions coming in well-defined intervals. What astonished me was the second hand on the big clock. The second hand would not move. I shut my eyes because sometimes time passes — a lot of time — if you shut your eyes. But that didn't work. Each second demanded its moment in the limelight, and there were sixty of them.

Did I ask for mercy?

I did.

Threshold? Forget threshold. I am becoming we. I thought I knew who I was, but now there are two of us and it will be that way for the rest of our lives.

"Move around," my sister says.

"I can't."

"Yes, move around. I'll hold you." My sister, Lynn, helps me stand. I hope every woman who ever gives birth has a sister with hands like my sister's hands. They are bigger than mine and stronger than mine, and she doesn't wear rings because she doesn't like to draw attention to them. She has quite a grip. She usually faints at the sight of blood, and there will be blood. What a grip she has.

I was there when Lynn gave birth to her daughter. I watched all the blood vessels break in Lynn's face because she was pushing so hard. Bright red dots all over her cheeks, as if someone had flicked the bristles of a wet paintbrush.

I remember wondering if the broken blood vessels in Lynn's face would heal, or would she be scarred for life? I found myself wanting to say, Is it really necessary to push *that* hard? But she seemed hell-bent on it.

I hope every woman who ever gives birth has somebody around with eyes like Steve's eyes.

Recently a friend of mine said she and her husband of twenty years were trying out a newfangled fancy kind of sex, and it was really good.

"Really, and how do you do it?"

"You just look in each other's eyes for the whole time and you don't look away no matter what and you don't shut your eyes no matter what. Try it," she said.

It's a method that also works for getting through contractions. Steve's eyes are big and blue, and they were locked on mine. He didn't look away. The second hand moved.

After sixteen hours a doctor walked into the room. She took a single glance at me from the foot of my bed, then my chart.

"Get her an epidural," she said. And she was gone. I wanted the epidural by then. I wanted it. I was tired. Even Steve and Lynn were tired. If we were watching the video we could fast-forward a few hours.

And pause.

The truth is, I have never looked at the video. I cannot look. There is my son's head, crowning. And a great wall of blood. Rewind. His heart rate is dropping. Push, push.

Lynn: "Lisa, listen, you have to push, okay? You really have to push."

"There he is, there he is. Is he okay? What's all that blood? Look at all the blood."

"We've got a problem here," the doctor said. "Is he breathing?"

"We've got a problem."

"Is it the scar? Doctor, is it the scar?"

"More epidural here. I'm going to have to reach in and touch the scar to see if it's torn. We'll have to wait ten minutes for the epidural."

"Is he breathing?"

Lynn: "Lisa, we have to let the doctors do their work."

And so there was a ten-minute interval while we waited for the second epidural to kick in and for the doctor to decide if I was bleeding to death. A team of doctors was working on Theo in the corner.

"He's breathing," they said.

Here is how the conversation went: Steve, I am going to die. No, you're not. Yes, Steve, I am. You're going to have to take care of this baby by yourself. No, I'm not. Yes, Steve, you are.

I let it hit me, the idea of bleeding to death. I looked it in the eye. The idea of the doctor reaching up inside me to touch the damaged scar.

Even the word *blood* can make me queasy since I gave birth to Theo. But the scar had not ruptured during his birth. It was only the placenta. The placenta had burst as soon as Theo's head was out. Perhaps it had attached itself to the scar in a weird way, who knows? What would have happened if it had burst before Theo's head was out? But it did not burst then and the scar did not tear and Theo arrived safe and sound in a river of blood.

There was an ambulance attendant standing in the corner of the room. They had asked my permission to have him witness the birth.

These guys need the experience, they'd said. The ambulance attendant stood in the gloom of an unlit corner. His chin was raised, his hands at his sides. He was like one of the guards at Buckingham Palace, stoic, rigid with vigilant attention. He's in the video, I'm pretty sure. I would like to say to him, Whoever you are, I love you. Thank you for staying in the corner keeping watch and remaining calm. And while I'm at it, thank you to every single person in that room for doing your job.

YESTERDAY WE WENT FOR a canoe ride in a lake deep in the woods. Steve paddled and I read *Harry Potter* to seven-year-old Theo. I had been reading for hours, my voice cracking and sore.

This was the last of the seven books. We've got about fifty pages left. Harry Potter is all grown up.

It is almost September and there's an autumn chill. Across the bay the spit of land that I have been trying to paint all summer is not emerald or lime green any more. It is tawny gold, with flares of rust. I am forty-three. I think I have an age spot on my right hand.

Okay, it might just be a big freckle, but I won't be having any more babies. I have a stepdaughter who is twenty-three, a daughter seventeen, and this blond boy in his bright orange life jacket, who demands I keep reading.

I loved being pregnant, every smell and colour. I loved how heavy my belly was. I loved sex and I loved my husband so much I felt cracked open by it. And I loved the smell of mown grass, dandelions screamingly yellow, the tug of the river over the hill from our house, all of the currents braiding together and unravelling.

I remember wanting my picture taken while I was very pregnant, near Archibald Falls. Climbing up on the rocks, the roar of water and the delicate rainbows hanging over the pool, and suddenly I was shaking with uncontrollable laughter, there on the side of the cliff, big and naked as an elephant, laughing so hard I could barely hang on to the slippery rocks, laughing so hard I was crying. I was on my hands and knees: joy is absurd. It is absurdly funny and humbling, and you happen upon it and all of life builds towards it and it doesn't last, and that's also funny: it doesn't last. Joy has a this-is-itness. And you can't remember it, not really, not accurately, when it's gone. There I was clinging to it. I had it in my fists and in my nostrils, I had it digging into my knees, it was falling on me in cold, shuddering curtains of mist.

I love the chaos of children: big messy paintings on newsprint and hula hoops, a tiara hanging on the banister, getting smacked in the head with a water balloon. I love galloping through the big epic. I can't believe it won't happen again.

But how demanding children are. They demand all of you, always, until there is nothing left of what you thought was you.

"Read on," Theo demands.

I am not having any more babies because it was too hard and dangerous for me, and the idea of it frightens me now, and I am in the middle of reading to Theo. But I miss being pregnant so much. I miss breastfeeding and diapers and I miss giving over and how humble that kind of love makes you, the love of a vulnerable being, and watching the dawn break because you've been awake all night, and the smell of cherry-flavoured cough syrup and high chairs, and I am afraid, very afraid, of the quiet and getting old, and I am glad for it.

FRANK

Leah McLaren

THE SECONDS THAT STRETCH between the act of giving birth and waiting to hear a baby cry are the most harrowing moments in an otherwise privileged life. My second son, Frank, didn't cry. Late last summer in a London hospital, he was born semi-conscious. His pulse was faint and he was floppy as a rag doll, a pale bluish grey in colour. There were angry red indents on his nose and skull that would later turn into deep purple bruises. According to his hospital notes his Apgar score at birth (on which 10 is hale and zero is non-responsive) was two.

Just before emerging, Frank turned to the left and got stuck in the birth canal—no amount of pushing could make him budge. He was wrenched out of me, first ineffectively with a vacuum and then later, definitively, with a pair of giant metal salad tongs called forceps. The midwife briefly placed his limp little body on my chest and then scooped him up again and over to the opposite side of the room where the doctors began their work.

At first, still dazed from the birth, I didn't fully understand what was going on. I remember thinking how strange it was that for hours on end all the focus had been on my body, and the monumental effort to make it do what it was supposed to, and now everything had shifted. It was like I'd been split in two and what was left of me — the remaining husk — seemed almost incidental to the scene.

I heard an alarm wailing in the corridor outside our room and I thought, vaguely, that there must be an emergency on this floor. Residents and interns in scrubs began streaming through the door, craning to see the patient — our motionless, minutes-old son. Before long there was a standing-room only crowd around the baby. My husband squeezed my hand as I processed the silent revelation that the emergency was us.

We watched the doctors placing a toy-sized oxygen mask on our son's face and heard them fall silent as their movements became quicker. We scanned their faces for panic or relief and saw nothing, only blankness. We waited for the baby's cry, but it never came.

Hours later, to our immense relief, we were told Frank was fine. The resident pediatrician made it clear he wasn't concerned — or even particularly interested — in Frank's case. He could offer no real explanation for why our son was born "flat-line" (his term) apart from the obvious deduction that he'd been knocked out by the grip of the forceps on his head. "It happens," the doctor said. "We don't know why." He had a touch of jaundice, but there had been no evidence of oxygen deprivation.

By contrast, I was worse for wear. In addition to the forceps, I'd had internal and external tearing as well as an episiotomy — cut open and stitched back together. As one doctor later put it: "It's like a truck drove through your pelvic floor." I was given transfusions for blood loss and paracetamol for the pain, which didn't help much.

When I was finally taken up to the neonatal unit in a wheelchair and able to hold him, my son was so bashed up he looked like he'd been in a bar fight. "You should see the other guy," the nurse joked. "You already have," I said. "The other guy is me."

This is not the story of a personal tragedy. I'm conscious while writing this of the many mothers who have experienced far worse. Pregnancy and childbirth, when it goes wrong, can result in all manner of horrors, including the loss of a child — an experience I cannot pretend to understand.

Instead, this is a story about what's been written out of Britain's official birth narrative. Frank's birth, as described, would be classified in our maternity system as a success. For a system that prides itself on being female-centred, the NHS maternity care system is failing post-natal women. Not only has the physical and mental health of new mothers become secondary, it sometimes seems inconsequential. This is the untold story of the suffering our maternity care system ignores.

It's difficult to admit this now, eight months after Frank's birth, but in those first weeks I did not feel the exhilaration that comes with a baby. I cared for my son dutifully, feeding, bathing, burping, swaddling, soothing him through the night, but much of the time I felt weirdly detached, like a zombie shuffling through the motions.

The sound of his cry induced black thoughts, a darkening of my already dull mood. I remember looking at him and registering the fact he was beautiful, but being unable to separate his body from the horror of his birth. I obsessed over the idea that something was wrong with him, that he'd been deprived of oxygen and the doctors had hidden it from me. I took him to see the community midwife twice because I was convinced his eyes were crossed. When I demanded to know if the midwife thought he looked like he had brain damage she looked at me oddly.

In those first few weeks I had flashbacks every day. I'd be standing in the queue at Sainsbury's and suddenly I'd be back in the madness of the delivery room, blood pooling on the floor beneath my bed wondering if my baby was dead. I ruminated over the details of what happened for weeks, unable to think about little else. Some days I told the story to anyone who would listen; others I could barely speak at all. Finally I went to see a psychiatrist who diagnosed me with trauma. Not post-partum depression—she was very clear on this point—but post-traumatic stress, as a result of the physical and emotional ordeal of Frank's birth.

Physically I was also struggling. As Frank grew bigger and bonnier, lighting up the world with his first gummy grins, I wasn't bouncing back. Every time I found myself alone in the room with a doctor, health visitor, or community midwife I'd demand they examine me to determine whether or not I was healing properly. Again and again I was told everything looked fine—the stitches had healed and I was given the all clear for exercise, for sex, for life. But something was amiss.

Like many new mothers I was suffering from stress incontinence (urinating when I coughed or sneezed) and a weakened pelvic floor, but there was something else. A strange dragging sensation, a heaviness that wouldn't abate. I described these symptoms over and over and was ignored by health professionals until one day, over a cup of tea, a girlfriend suggested I might be suffering from a pelvic organ prolapse. The next day I booked an appointment with my GP, who referred me to a gynecologist, who confirmed that, indeed, I had a moderate-to-severe case of a condition called cystocele, otherwise known as a prolapse of the bladder. What this means is that my vaginal wall was so badly damaged giving birth that my bladder was spilling out into my vagina. The best course of treatment, he told me, was corrective surgery. It's something I can't have until I'm three months clear of breastfeeding, which is some months away yet. In the meantime I've been prescribed a course of post-natal physiotherapy, which involves performing pelvic floor exercises under the supervision of a doctor and having vibrating wands shoved up my nether regions in order to reverse tissue damage.

This is not as fun as it sounds.

In spite of all this, I'm one of the lucky ones. Most women who experience birth injury and trauma never get properly diagnosed or treated. It's hard even to get anyone to recognize there might be a problem. My husband, astonished there was no routine follow-up for me after such a traumatic birth, tracked down the obstetrician who'd delivered Frank to seek guidance from her. She did not respond. We found out later this sort of contact is not encouraged; no comment or advice could be offered. A hospital collectively delivers.

The Birth Trauma Association, a peer-to-peer support group, estimates that 10,000 women in Britain are treated for post-traumatic stress disorder as a result of birth each year. That's the largest single cohort of PTSD sufferers in the country. They estimate as many as 200,000 more women may feel traumatized by childbirth and develop untreated symptoms of PTSD.

On the physical injury side, the *British Journal of Obstetrics and Gynaecology* in 2015 found that 24 percent of women still experience pain during sex eighteen months after giving birth. The same year researchers from the University of Michigan gave sixty-eight women MRIS seven weeks after having babies. Of the admittedly small sample, they found 29 percent had fractures in their pubic bones, which all of them were unaware of, and 41 percent had tearing and severe damage to their pelvic floor muscles that had remained undiagnosed. Another recent U.S. study, published in the journal PLOS One, found 77 percent of mothers still suffered from back pain and 49 percent experienced urinary incontinence a year after having their babies.

It's obvious that childbirth is deeply traumatic for many women's minds and bodies. Just over a century ago almost 7 percent of pregnant women in England and Wales died from it. But birth is much safer now — so why are so many women still suffering its after-effects undiagnosed and untreated?

Part of the reason is that the conversation around birth trauma and injury is steeped in shame and institutional sexism. I'm not just talking about the general prudishness surrounding women's reproductive health issues. There is a prevailing attitude I encountered among many health professionals which is that new mothers should basically learn to suck it up. As one GP said to me in semi-exasperation: "You've had two children. Your body's changed. You can't expect to feel the same as you did before."

Rebecca Schiller, chair of BirthRights, an organization that seeks to promote human rights in childbirth, told me that institutional denial of women's experience is a huge problem, especially when it comes to post-natal care. "There is a general attitude of 'Your experience doesn't matter, all that matters is a healthy baby.'" When, of course, the two are inextricably related.

Part of the problem, I have come to believe, is that pregnant women are not properly informed of the risks of birth trauma and injury in advance.

With my first pregnancy I was determined to have an all-natural, drug-free, at-home water birth. I rented a birth pool at the urging of my NHS homebirth midwife and when labour began I went around the house lighting scented candles. But seven hours in, when my baby turned out to be an undetected breech, I was rushed to hospital in a wailing ambulance. Once it was determined my son would be born via emergency Caesarean, a doctor talked me through all the risks in advance and asked me to sign a surgical waiver. And yet, with my second son, when I waived my right to an elective C-section and opted instead for a "normal" birth, I was assured by several midwives that opting for a VBAC (vaginal birth after Caesarean) was the safer, better option and would result in an easier recovery than a surgical birth.

As I found out later, women in my age group (forty), especially those who have had a previous C-section, have much higher rates of assisted births—and assisted births often lead to injury and trauma. The NHS and the NCT have very little to say on birth trauma. There are no birth trauma or injury counselling services and after care, as I found out, is difficult to come by. There are private options (like my psychiatrist), but there are private options for everything if you can afford it.

To get state-funded care, you have to fight for it, which many birth-injured and traumatized new mothers are in no state to do. Complicating matters further is the issue of post-partum depression. Just look at the post-natal chat groups online and you will find women frustrated at being told they simply have a hormonally induced case of "baby blues" when what they're actually feeling is a normal reaction to a profoundly distressing experience. Diagnosing a birth-injured or traumatized mother with post-partum depression is the healthcare equivalent of asking a justifiably irate woman if maybe, just maybe, she's about to get her period? And yet it happens all the time.

There is a reasonable explanation for this apparent state of institutional denial. Birth trauma and injury conflict with the NHS's dominant maternity care ethos, that "natural" births are safer and more empowering for women. This despite the fact that the U.K. has one of the highest infant mortality rates in western Europe and, according to the NHS litigation authority, pays out hundreds of millions in maternity negligence claims each year.

As the NHS continues to pay scant attention to the issue, rates of birth injury and trauma continue to rise, due to a confluence of factors including ageing mothers, obesity and larger newborns. But why isn't more attention paid to the routine psychological and physical harm endured by so many post-natal woman?

This is a question Maureen Treadwell, chair of the Birth Trauma Association, has been asking for nearly two decades. She founded her organization in response to the number of women she knew who'd been refused pain relief during labour and ended up traumatized by the experience. "If a man underwent dental surgery having begged for anesthetic and not received any, we'd recommend therapy — yet if the same thing happens to a woman we tell her she's a good girl, well done. It's madness," she said.

According to Treadwell, birth trauma is exacerbated by a culture that celebrates only one kind of birth. "The system, as well as the dominant culture, fills women with false expectations. It deludes women into thinking that birth ought to be this wonderful, empowering experience and when it isn't women feel terribly ashamed."

Last year when Jamie and Jools Oliver had their fifth child, Oliver tweeted about his wife's "unbelievably composed natural birth." It sounds ridiculous, but I cried reading that tweet. New mothers are deeply susceptible to guilt and it often begins with not having performed birth in the circumscribed way.

Eight months on, Frank and I are muddling along in an exhausted state of contentment. The trauma of his birth is fading, superseded each passing day with the marvellous reality of him. My body is now the body of a mother—battle-worn, cozy, and intimidating in its accomplishments. I am grateful for my boys and for the fact that I got help for a condition many mothers experience but for which few ever seek acknowledgement, let alone treatment.

Like I said, I'm one of the lucky ones.

FLIGHT OF THE WENDYBIRD

Lynn Coady

We all live in a capital I
In the middle of the desert
In the center of the sky
—Sesame Street

WHAT IS THAT THING God said in the Bible? I am alpha and omega. The first and the last, the beginning and the end. I'm like that too, on a smaller scale. I am my own beginning, middle, and end. That is, there is nothing on either side of me. I was some-one's child, someone else was my child. But I don't know either of those people I just mentioned, and likely never will. One I met very briefly, but neither of them are in my life. They exist, but I don't have to believe in them if I don't want to.

Lots of people in versions of my situation will choose to do just that—to disbelieve. To behave as if these individuals, whose bodies are so intricately, inexorably connected to your own, don't exist. No one minds if you decide to do this, but strangely enough, plenty of people mind if you decide to do the opposite. I've never understood that. Can you imagine if your sister or someone just announced to everyone, say, at Thanksgiving dinner, "I've decided I don't believe in Cousin Waldo anymore." And everyone at the table just nodded and murmured, "Yes, yes. That's probably for the best."

I just wrote a thing. Actually, I didn't write it just now; I was going over the first few pages of a novel I recently wrote about Adoption. (I write Adoption with a capital A in order to get at its institutional underpinnings. Because I'm not talking about adoption of a fake French accent or a polluted stretch of highway, after all. I'm talking about the legal contortions our society has developed to allow for the exchange of children, i.e., humans.)

Anyway, I wrote this thing about the Wendybird in *Peter Pan*. Do you remember the Wendybird? That's what they called Wendy at first, before they knew who she was. More specifically, that's how the homicidal fairy Tinkerbell identified her to the credulous Lost Boys.

"Shoot her down!" exhorted the psychopathic fairy. "Kill the Wendybird!"

"All right, we will," said the obedient Lost Boys.

In my book, my character, an adoptee named Wendy, considers this incident. Her mother has named her Wendy because the mother imagined her adopted daughter, pre-adoption, to be like the Lost Boys in *Peter Pan*—"wild and alone." So she wants to name her daughter after the Lost Boys, but Wendy is a girl, so her mother names her Wendy.

My Wendy thinks, But Wendy wasn't a Lost Boy. She was a mother. That's how she's presented in J. M. Barrie's tale, a breast-less, ringleted mother who can't stand the thought of all those innocent children being alone and uncared for in Never-Never

Land. So she rushes after Peter Pan in order to be by their sides and make everything better in their lives.

And the Lost Boys shot her down. That's the line I was thinking about today. I was tweaking it, as we say in the writing business. I tweaked the line and something became clear to me. I'd thought I'd been making some kind of metaphorical point about my character Wendy and how, during the course of the novel, she would be emotionally "shot down" in some way or another (I know, I know: deep!). But as I tweaked the line, the real meaning took shape. I realized I wasn't talking about the Wendy in my story at all. I was talking about the Mother.

And note that I'm capitalizing that one too.

The Mother was doomed; that was the point of the Wendybird anecdote. The Mother was well meaning and only wanted to do the right thing. She wanted to swoop to the side of the dear little children. She wanted to be their salvation. The Mother was doomed. Birth mother, adopted mother, mother mother. The Mother is always shot down.

CONSIDER THE ABOVE a storyteller's clearing of the throat. An opera singer's vocal warm-ups: *me-me-me-meeee!* That was the story's prologue. Here is what I've always thought of as its beginning.

Me and my brother Jimmy are driving around in a truck. I'm happy, because Jimmy is paying attention to me. He has taken me to A&W and bought me a Whistle Dog. He doesn't often do this sort of thing now that he's in university. We all look up to Jimmy. He's not doing so well in university, is behaving a little recklessly, but nobody in my family knows that yet. He is the oldest brother, and therefore King of the Siblings. In my parents' eyes he still can do no wrong.

I eat my Whistle Dog and now I'm bouncing around in the truck, sipping on a diet root beer. We're just driving around now, and Jimmy starts talking.

"When guys say they're going to stop," he tells me, "don't believe them. They're not going to stop."

I take a pensive sip of root beer. This is wonderful. Apparently I've become so cool and grown-up in the last little while that Jimmy has deemed it appropriate to discuss sex with me, just as I've heard him do with his buddies over the past few years before yelling at me to get out from behind the couch or put down the phone extension. I feel like I've leapt some kind of adolescent hurdle.

"Huh!" I say, easing into the topic as casually as Jimmy has initiated it. "They won't?"

"Fuck, no," says Jimmy. "A guy's not going to stop in the middle of the greatest feeling of his life!"

Despite the seen-it-all demeanour I'm struggling to affect, this formulation gives me pause. The greatest feeling of his life? *Really?* But I don't interrogate further, as this kind of thing is clearly common knowledge in Jimmy's circle.

Jimmy steers the truck up a dirt road where he can really open 'er up. He's always enjoyed speeding, which will get him into some trouble in the impending years.

"It's best to do it just after your oil change," adds Jimmy, swerving the truck a little for my entertainment.

"Is it?" I place a hand on the dashboard to brace myself, tittering.

"Yeah. And get him to wear a condom. He'll do it. You might not think he will, but he will. If you say, 'Fuck you, get a condom or no deal,' he'll do it."

"Okay," I say, coming down off my high a little. Jimmy,

I realize at the mention of condoms, is acting on my parents' behalf. From the moment I turned fifteen I've been treated—for reasons I am only beginning to fathom—like some sort of walking affront to Christian decency.

I might add, this is a tense period in general where my family is concerned. Money is extremely tight. I don't really understand that because I don't understand money, but I feel it every day in my nerve endings. My two older brothers are in university, and their loans cover only so much. Both my parents are working. When I am not at school, a paid housekeeper looks after my invalid grandmother. My job is to relieve the housekeeper at 3:30 p.m. sharp.

When my mother and father come home from work, with Uncle Larry in tow from his day at the special school, I will have spent the past two and a half hours listening for my grandmother and fending off my little brother, who wants to play and do something fun, whereas I only want to lie on the couch. At this time in our lives there are a lot of people in the house who need looking after.

Dad typically arrives home enraged by something Uncle Larry has done to provoke him on the drive home, like asking why the car is stopping every time they come to a stop sign and exhorting, "Come on, come on, come on!" until they get moving again. Sometimes when things are particularly frantic, we have to get a local cab man to take Larry home. He tried out the stop-sign trick a few times on one of them before the driver pulled over, got out of the front seat, and climbed into the back beside my uncle. "You drive the fucking car," he told Larry, folding his arms. This story kept my father in stitches for months.

The point is, though, Dad usually arrives home in rage, and Larry in tears. And the tears enrage my father more, because they make it seem like he is a bad man who yells at his handicapped brother as opposed to a good man who is taking care of his handicapped brother and aged mother at considerable personal cost. And nobody seems to goddamn appreciate it! And so there is yelling.

So my days take shape in a fog of anxiety and depression. I hate every single moment of school. I come home with migraines, as exhausted and soul-weary as your average underpaid office drone. I am yelled at in the morning when I get up, and every night before I go to bed.

I don't characterize my life in this way at the time—as a depressive fog. For all I know, this is what life is.

But you can see why I would want to go out with my friends and get piss-loaded drunk as often as humanly possible.

My parents have started leaving pamphlets from church on my bed about the dangers of premarital sex. Apparently it leads one to get pregnant, and diseased, and to be a diseased and pregnant slut. The aimless truck ride with Jimmy, I realize, is the second wave.

Which is too bad, because it would be nice to just be driving around drinking root beer with Jimmy for no good reason at all—just because he likes my company. But no, it's due to the psychic terror I lately inspire in my parents. I feel tired realizing this, but still pretty engaged by the conversation. After all, how often does your older brother talk to you about sex? How often does anyone, except the pamphlets?

"But never do it just before your oil change," my brother continues.

"Okay," I say.

We speak of other things for a while. Jimmy regales me with a piquant anecdote or two from his own sexual history, and I hang

on every word. Finally I screw up my courage and wait for a lull
in the conversation.

I ask my brother, as lightly, as casually as I'm able, "What's
an oil change?"

He turns to look at me for the first time during our conversation. Just a touch of my parents' holy terror colours his expression. "Your *period*, for God's sake! Your period! Jesus Christ! You
didn't know what I was talking about this whole time?"

I laugh and laugh. Who calls it an oil change?

THAT WAS CAPE BRETON in 1986.

Here is the story's middle. I am throwing up. I am more tired
than I have ever been. In class I can't keep my head up. There is
a sickroom adjoining the principal's office, and I ask to go in and
lie down. I miss two classes in a row and wake up with no idea
what time it is.

I think I am getting a beer belly, so I join the gym at the
Wandalyn Inn.

We Catholic girls head out to Mass together. Me and Lise
and Nicole and Christine. Lise is driving her parents' car. A girl
who lives two houses up the street from me has recently been
revealed to be pregnant. The news hit the town like a stink bomb.
This is huge. This is explosive. We talk about it endlessly. What
would you do? Christine asks from the front seat. Would you
have an abortion?

The funny thing is, we all talk as if this is something we could
just go and do. Like we'd just haul out the Yellow Pages and dial
an 800 number.

"I could never do that," says Nicole, the rote response.

"I'd kill myself!" I tell them sunnily.

I go to a doctor who is not my family doctor. He places a hand on my abdomen. It takes him less than a minute to make his diagnosis—just touching me like that, like some kind magician or faith healer. But instead of proclaiming, "Healed!" he says, "Oh dear, I think you're pregnant."

I go to another doctor, this time with my boyfriend. I need to find someone who will understand intuitively what has to be done. But I've forgotten my health card. I'm only seventeen, I'm used to my family doctor, I don't know about these things. So the doctor just yells at me for not bringing my health card. I sit there dripping snot and tears all over myself because I haven't got any Kleenex. I'm always getting yelled at. The boyfriend has occasionally taken his turn, but he doesn't today. He's nice to me as we sit on the steps outside the doctor's office, trying to clean me up.

We go to a movie in Antigonish with Lise and John. You want irony? It's *For Keeps*, with Molly Ringwald. A teenage girl gets pregnant. She and her boyfriend get married. They have a baby. They love the baby. They have some difficult times, but it all works out in the end.

Afterwards I become violently ill. I sit on the curb, vomiting helplessly into a storm drain.

"Don't look at me," I tell my boyfriend, who is watching me just as helplessly.

There is one more doctor left in town, who happens to live directly across the street from Lise. I've babysat for this doctor a couple of times. She is the wife of a local politician. We knock on her door, because that's the kind of thing you can do in my town. Just go to a doctor's house at night and knock on the door.

She is kind, gives me an anti-nauseant, and tells me to come to her office the next day.

"I'd like an abortion," I tell her the next day.

I know this doctor, I know the politician husband. They are

as Catholic as John Paul II. I know what she's going to say. But in the doctor's defence, things are pretty far along at this point. The first trimester is almost at an end.

"I just don't think it would be good for you," she tells me. I believe her. I still believe her.

Later she will give me her old maternity clothes.

I STILL OWN THE MATERNITY clothes I was wearing the day I went into labour. They are in my closet. I could go pull them out and put them on and sit here wearing them if I wanted. That was nineteen years ago — more years than I'd been alive at that point. I was wearing a pink button-down shirt of the doctor's, which I liked very much, and a pair of black pants with an elastic waistband from Cotton Ginny.

I don't know how or when it happened, but at some point I turned to steel. Or maybe that's not it. I just decided, *Here's what's going to happen.*

What is going to happen is this: none of the things people seem to think should happen, that's for sure.

I am not going to go stay with the nuns. This is my dad's idea. It's like from the turn of the century or something.

I am not going to marry my boyfriend. This was never the plan; why should it be now?

I am not going to stay in Cape Breton and keep it and live with my parents and work at Dairy Queen and be a stereotype. I'm already enough of a stereotype as it is.

I'm not going to put off going to university.

Here's what's going to happen. I'm going to Ottawa for the rest of the summer. I'll stay at a home for unwed mothers (Oh God help me, this was my own turn-of-the-century mindset. I'd stay at a home for unwed mothers, sure). I know that once I get to Ottawa I will be welcome to stay with my beloved Aunt Helen, but I don't want to do that. I want to be alone. I want to do this alone. I have a conviction that this is the definitive moment of my adulthood, and it threatens to overwhelm and dominate me forever, so I am grabbing it by the horns and wrestling it to the ground and sticking knives in it. If I were a man I'd call this an assertion of my manhood. But *womanhood* doesn't have the same connotations. When your anatomy defies your will and you decide you are going to by Christ smack it into submission, you don't call that an assertion of womanhood. I don't know what you call that.

I am due mid-September. I will put off moving into university residence until after the blessed event. Meanwhile I will contact social services about Adoption.

To sum up, I'll have it, I'll give it away, I'll start school, and everything will be fine.

All the girls at the Salvation Army home for unwed mothers are stupid sluts. I am not stupid, or a slut. Well, okay, maybe there's no getting around the slut thing at this juncture. But I'm not stupid. My roommate runs her hair dryer at seven in the morning while I'm sleeping. Later she tells me I shouldn't pluck my eyebrows because God meant for that hair to be there.

"Do you shave your legs?" I ask her. She stands with her mouth open. Stupid slut, I think, turning back to the mirror.

Cheryl and I walk down the street to the corner store. She complains about men constantly harassing her. In fact, it is happening right now.

"See?" she says.

Cheryl, I sigh to myself. *Your boobs are enormous and you swathe them in spandex, you stupid slut.*

Why do I hate these stupid sluts? Because they terrify me,

and it feels better to name them as I do in my mind. That's the easiest thing to call them. In fact they are helpless girls with no money who are going to have babies and have been rejected by their families and have no idea what to do now.

But I don't regret being here. I don't ask myself why I don't go to Aunt Helen's, where I'll be loved and cared for, thus freeing up a bed for some girl who doesn't have that option. I'm not going anywhere. I'm doing this alone.

I've been going to the university on the bus every day to organize things for my classes, to get my student ID, to make arrangements to move into residence at the end of September.

It's September now. I've never been all that big, but I'm starting to feel it—a certain awkward girth, a heaviness. But I'm still as small as ever—if you saw me on the street, you wouldn't know I was pregnant.

"My goodness," says the obstetrics nurse. "You're certainly keeping things packed all nice and neat in there."

It's mid-September. My mother wants to fly out when the time comes.

"How are you doing?" she asks me on the phone. "Anything?" I am thinking about a science project Jimmy did when we were kids. He hatched chickens in a Styrofoam cooler set up in our living room. One of the embryos he even managed to remove from the egg and transfer into a glass jar. He kept it warm, just as he did the eggs, and eventually the thing in the jar started pecking to get out. We just sat there and watched it pecking eternally against the glass.

"Nope," I say. "Nothing." I'm weirdly proud of this. Maybe nothing will ever happen. It will live inside me like a chicken in a jar.

"Okay," says Mom, hanging up with kissing noises.

She calls back an hour later. "Oh, to hell with it," she tells me. "I'm flying out tomorrow."

Woman's intuition. The day after she arrives we are supposed to go shopping (the other girls in the Sally Ann home have no idea what to make of me at this point. Her *mother* is taking her *shopping?*). When she arrives to pick me up, I am in the upstairs bathroom, where I've sequestered myself for reasons of privacy. I seem to be constipated. I'm in there for an hour. When I emerge, it turns out the whole house has been looking for me.

"It could be labour," says one of the staff.

"No, no," I assure them. "I just really have to go to the bathroom."

"Maybe we should just go and get you checked out," suggests my mother.

The maternity hospital is right next door, so we simply stroll down the street. I'm thinking how embarrassing this is going to be. What if they want to give me an enema? This whole pregnancy thing has required a steady denuding of my physical dignity. Once, during an examination, a whole team of medical students stood gawping while the doctor fidgeted around in my vaginal canal. Meanwhile I stared up at a cartoon pasted to the ceiling that featured a woman in a public bathroom with one leg hoisted in the air. She was using the automatic hand dryer in order to dry herself after having a pee. I laughed despite myself, with all the med students gathered around. Dignity, schmignity, the cartoon seemed to be saying.

"You're in labour," says the nurse.

"No," I say.

They admit me.

Let's stop now. I've changed my mind. Probably I just need an enema. I almost suggest this to the professionals scuttling around me. I'd cheerfully submit to an enema at this point.

I drink some chocolate milk and vomit it up a moment later. The nurses clean me up with insect-like efficiency. They roll me to and fro on the bed as they change the sheets. It's like being on a boat.

Someone checks between my legs.

"Whoa!" she says. "You've really dilated in the last hour."

It seems to me this shouldn't be happening quite so fast. On TV, women scream and moan and they do that TV time-passing trick to let you know that hours and hours have gone by, and everyone involved looks exhausted and bedraggled. I'm fresh as a daisy. I can't have been here for more than two hours — three, tops — and for the most part things haven't been too bad. The nurses have even marvelled at how quiet and agreeable I've been, except for the throwing up. My mother tells them I was like that when I was a baby too. I never cried. Whenever I'm expected to be crying and kicking up a fuss, I never do it. I keep things packed all nice and neat in there.

"Uh-oh," I say. A flood has occurred between my legs.

The nurses re-enact their insect cleaning routine, cracking wise about Niagara Falls.

A doctor, who introduced himself to me when I was admitted, now reappears.

"Now's the time to decide if you want an epidural," he says.

"What's an epidural?" I ask.

"We freeze your spine."

"I don't know," I say. I look to my mother. "Do I need an epidural?"

"When you're completely dilated," explains the doctor. "That's when the labour will really kick in."

"You mean it will hurt?"

"Well," he says, "it could be very intense. But you have to decide now, or it'll be too late to give you one."

I think about all the screaming and moaning on television.

"Okay," I say. "I'll have one."

They stick a needle into my spine and my eyes almost *sproing*, cartoon-like, out of my head. It feels absolutely, incontrovertibly *wrong*, a needle in the spine.

"She's completely dilated," says a nurse a moment or two later.

"Oh no!" I say. Too soon, too soon.

They roll me into the delivery room.

"Mommy!" I say. Or it could be I just think that. My mother is right there in any case.

The doctor was right—this is where the labour really kicks in. But he lied about the epidural because this experience is very intense. He said it could be very intense without it, but it is very intense with it as well. I wonder what it would have been like if they hadn't shoved the needle in my spine. Screaming, I suppose, instead of just moaning, which is what I'm doing now. A description of childbirth, which I gleaned from a Jackie Collins novel of all places, flits through my mind: *like shitting a football*.

"Can't you just take it out?" I say after a while.

"No, because you have to push."

"But I think it's *stuck* there."

"You have to push."

So I push.

"I see the head," says someone.

Oh, come on, I want to say. You do not. What a cliché this whole thing is.

Then a kind of internal physical popping sensation takes place down there, and I know intuitively what has happened.

The shoulders have worked their way out. And something slithers away from me.

"*Waah*," complains the person.

"I'm *sorry*," I say.

THAT WAS THE STORY'S middle. This is how it more or less ends. A nurse approaches my bedside later on. She is very nice. She wants me to know what an extraordinarily easy delivery I had. Child-bearing hips. Apparently I've got hips like the Champs Élysées. She tells me that one day, when I meet that "special guy" I want to have all sorts of babies with, I should have no problems at all.

"It's like you were made for it," she tells me.

This is not at all what I want to hear.

I want her to tell me, This is actually all fine. This is going to be easy. I know it doesn't seem fine, or easy, right now. It has very recently revealed itself to you as a grotesque distortion of how the world should be. It has very recently revealed itself to you as an obscene nightmare. You have recently come to understand that this nightmare is going to constitute your reality for a very long time. If I may quote Joyce, for we maternity nurses are hugely into modernist literature, this will be a nightmare from which you can't awake. Oh, I know how laughable it all seems now. How laughable a formulation: *I'll have it, I'll give it away. Simple!* And everyone will do what they can to make it seem simple. This lie will only add to the monstrosity. The monstrosity is quite complex. It will take on layers, shades, and colours over the years. It will distort. Sometimes it will seem more benign than others, but most times it will only seem like what it is: awfulness, perpetually transforming, perpetually taking on nuance. Just when you think it's retreating: *pow!* It merely camouflaged itself in order to surprise you. It's tricky! It's playful that way! Here it is again, and it's all new! improved! in living colour! It doesn't go away. It makes the world a different hue—there's a before hue and an after hue, and it can never go back to what it was before. You begin to see jokes where no one else sees jokes. You see perversity where no one else sees perversity. You, therefore, are perverse. So you become the creature you will be, not the person you had planned. And as you live, side by side with the monstrosity, so do you become monstrous yourself. Because really, it's not a question of side by side at all. It's in your body and of your body—it *is* your body, and it's never going anywhere.

In a way, of course, it's exactly what you wanted: Garbo. Capital I.

But you don't have to worry about any of that, continues the kindly nurse. This is actually all fine. This is going to be easy.

THE ROAD TO HECTANOOGA

Christy Ann Conlin

REMEMBERING MY SON'S BIRTH is not something I do often, not in detail. It was the singularly most painful occurrence of my life. I have a quiet worry that if I delve too deeply the pain will spring forth like a panther waiting in the night. And yet when I do remember, the pain—the visceral, throbbing agony—has receded. I remember my face contorted in the bathroom mirror, and in that reflection I see suffering but I do not feel it. I trace only the memory of it. It is this absolute transformation of memory that astounds me. I am nothing but biology, my chemistry acting on mind and emotion, my very recall of the most important experience of my life altered. I am left remembering the memory of a great pain that gave me my son.

We have a birth video, and although Silas has just turned two, I've never watched it. We have a birth story written by Alice, our doula, but until the past few days I had never read it. Two leaves are glued onto the front page, leaves she collected on a walk we took that autumn day when I was in labour. We have photos of the birth, and I'm always shocked by the absolute exhaustion in my face, the despair, my eyes full of suffering. I think it was at around hour twenty-five of my twenty-nine-hour labour that I asked for a lobotomy. I had already asked for an epidural—and been denied. I recall a scorching sense of outrage when they said it was too late—too late for an epidural, not a lobotomy. Those weren't routine, they said. I couldn't have one of those. All our careful preparations and no one had said there was a point of no return, that there was an epidural cut-off point. It would slow things down, they told me. It might result in other interventions. Just push, they said. I remember the sense of betrayal rising out of me like an animal. Then a sense of absolute helplessness. I wanted a general anesthetic and a Caesarean section. I could go on no more.

I think someone laughed.

"Push," they all said. I remember that.

"Push," said the obstetrician.

"Push," said the doula, my partner, James, and our dear friend Gwen.

And good old Nurse Carrie.

"Push-push-push."

Push them out the window, I thought.

Push-push-push this amazing pressure out from between my legs. Then I think I fell asleep. I was so tired. I fell asleep between those last contractions. Waking, panicking when one would come and Alice wasn't at my side. I do remember pushing, but now I can't remember the pain except as in a dream, a soft anguish that undulates in my mind's eye like a moon jellyfish, delicate and translucent edges rippling and waving into darkness. They call it disassociative amnesia. The disruption of a memory. It's a symptom of post-traumatic stress disorder. Apparently you can have this experience at some point after childbirth. Not PTSD (although I'm more than sure after my own excruciating, twenty-nine-hour, non-medicated labour that birthing causes both diagnosed and undiagnosed PTSD), but disassociative amnesia, when the memory of the birthing becomes muted and soft, less precise. When parts disappear altogether. Holes. When the gushes of fluid and blood, the straining and gasping, my fingernails cutting into James's palms, his face so helpless and tired as I strained to push this new life out of me, when all of these memories became so many silk prayer flags, each imprinted with a story, a recollection, fluttering and falling endlessly in my mind. And the creature waving the prayer flags is of course biology, softening the memories to ensure that a woman will go through that exquisite agony once more lest the species die out.

I WAS THIRTY-NINE WHEN SILAS was conceived and forty when I gave birth. Through all the relationships I'd had, the veritable chocolate box of boyfriends and lovers I'd devoured, I'd not ever met someone I desired to have a child with. And that's what I wanted in the realm of babies and families, to have a child in partnership with a man I truly loved. When I was thirty-five I moved back to Nova Scotia from Northern Ireland, where I had been on my latest sojourn. I had just sold my first novel, and I wanted to base myself back home in Nova Scotia, in the Annapolis Valley near the Bay of Fundy. It was at this time that a friend, an ex-lover and physician I'd stayed in touch with, pointed out to me that I was thirty-five, and if I wanted to have children I should probably start thinking seriously about it, because at thirty-five a woman's fertility begins an unavoidable plunge down a long and inevitable cliff. He was shocked at my naïveté. How could an educated and intelligent woman not know this?

I was shocked as well. Why didn't I know this? How could

it be? I'd spent my life chasing all sorts of dreams but not the baby one. I hadn't known my fertility would decline. I thought I'd eventually meet Mr. Right and it would all fall into place. In the meantime I'd do all the things I loved. But that's the problem with assumptions. And that's the problem with theoretical desires and abstract longings. Yes, sure, I wanted children. But my passion was seeing the world, and this was where my energy went, my focus and my effort. Having kids was like buying a house—something I wanted to do way down the road. And then somehow during my travels I found writing, and writing became my biggest passion, the love of my life.

But I came to writing late. I didn't take up the pen—or in the contemporary manifestation, put fingers to the keyboard—until I was thirty. And then writing consumed me, until I met James when I was selling daffodils for the Canadian Cancer Society. I was working on my second novel and living on an apple farm on the South Mountain, overlooking the Annapolis Valley. James and I had worked together as kids on his family strawberry farm. I hadn't seen him in years. When we did meet, we had an instant connection, or reconnection, as it were. We were drawn together by a common history, a shared love of Nova Scotia and the rocky shores of the Bay of Fundy, of fishing in the spring, of pussy willows and mayflowers and the moon in the sky in all its manifestations. James has two daughters, Mary and Anna, from a previous relationship, and it was seeing him with them, seeing the tender vulnerability in parenting, that moved me in a unique way and finally made my desire to have a baby tangible, palpable. We decided to have a child together.

AT THE FETAL ASSESSMENT Clinic at the IWK Health Centre in Halifax I was called AMA—*advanced maternal age*. The clinic deals with mothers who are at risk for a wide variety of reasons, among them having a baby at the age of thirty-five or older. There were all kinds of potential chromosomal complications, given my old, withered eggs. I was attended to by a bevy of maternal/fetal medicine physicians who performed a battery of tests, all to determine our risk of having a baby with a veritable cornucopia of deformities and abnormalities. I'd been pregnant the year before, but at fourteen weeks they couldn't detect a heartbeat. They thought I might have a molar pregnancy. I remember lying on the table in the ultrasound room, the specialist calling in another specialist, an older man who spoke to me in clinical terms. *A molar pregnancy isn't really a pregnancy. Rather than a fetus, it is an abnormal tissue mass, placental tissue, a hydatidiform mole. In some cases a molar pregnancy can result in gestational trophoblastic disease. And a small percentage of these cases become cancerous.* He pointed at the ultrasound screen. *From the mass in the uterus, we think you might in fact have a hydatidiform mole.*

I can't remember what else he said. I know he kept talking. I asked him to leave me, and with a soft nod and a gentle pat on my arm he did, and then it was just me and the ultrasound screen.

I was scheduled for a D & C the next day. And then I had to wait for the pathology report. The report wasn't conclusive, so it was sent away for a second opinion. If ever there was a moment where my fertility seemed to be drying up in my hands, crumbling and turning to dust and falling from my fingertips, it was then. Why had I waited so long? Why hadn't having a baby been my burning desire when I was younger, when it was easier and not so fraught with complications? With my face pressed against the brick wall in the hospital hall, my fingernails in front of my eyes, dirty nails like those of a child, I cried.

But I hadn't had a molar pregnancy. Instead I had had a missed miscarriage, which is when you lose the pregnancy but the body doesn't naturally expel it. I hadn't realized how many women have miscarriages for no discernable reason. How many women have miscarriages who go on to have healthy babies. But still, for our second pregnancy I was nervous. We conceived a month after the D & C. There was no problem with fertility. The ultrasound was normal and the baby seemed healthy. And my test results gave me the same chance as a healthy eighteen-year-old of having a baby with a genetic problem. But after my first experience, I was apprehensive. I was holding my breath for the first six months.

My pregnancy was a joyous time once we arrived at the heart of the second trimester. We had our nifty doula, Alice, and she was guiding us through the experience. Alice is a tiny woman from Newfoundland who now lives on the North Mountain in a big house in the woods with her two sons. She is confident and grounded about birthing, so knowledgeable and calm, always light and humorous. Her greatest gift to us during the pregnancy was putting us at ease. There wasn't anything Alice couldn't manage. I glowed. I was radiant. I had stylish maternity clothes. I had boundless energy and worked constantly on my novel. I would be pregnant forever. It would go on like the ocean, like infinity.

And I didn't spend much time thinking about its end, when I would go into labour, when the baby would be born. People were eager to share their stories, both men and women. But there was no continuity to the stories except in the way they were offered, cradled in the tender arms of the tellers, offering a glimpse of this moment in time that had changed their lives forever. These stories were all different. Some went into great detail and some revealed only bits and pieces, and I found the endless range of experience alarming. I had no idea what to expect. I'd ask questions, but even the answers confused me. One of my best friends told me to get an epidural, to bypass the pain from the onset.

"What pain?" I asked her. "Is it that bad?"

"I don't know," she said. "I was medicated."

And so I stopped asking people about their birth stories, though with my enormous belly leading the way, people didn't stop sharing them. I didn't read many birth stories either. Perhaps it was the lingering worry from the failed first pregnancy. I couldn't conceive of a human being bursting out of me, and thinking about it was unnerving. It was beyond my comprehension.

My friend Millie was telling me a story when I was in the ninth month of pregnancy. It was about the interminable drive her parents would take her on to see her Acadian grandparents back in the sixties. They'd drive down to the French Shore and then turn inland from the ocean on the long way to Hectanooga. Her father always drove at the speed limit on that old, bumpy road, not one notch over. I interrupted. What was it like when you had your kids? She has two children and three grandchildren, and a great grandchild on the way.

And these are the wisest words I was offered: *You'll know soon enough. You'll know. You have to go through it to understand. It's always different. It will be what it is and then you can tell me. It's the same as the drive to see my grandparents—you'd have to be in that car to understand that it was always a long old drive to Hectanooga.*

WE'D PREPARED FOR THE stages of birth with Alice. She brought a doll over and a pelvis made of foam, and she showed James and me and the girls how the head would come into the birth canal. The girls would take the foam pelvis and wear it as a hat. Alice asked me if I'd heard of the ring of fire. "No," I said. "Well," she said, "that's something you might feel when the baby's head starts to come out." I didn't want to think about that, although I had Johnny Cash lurking about in my head for the rest of the pregnancy. I'd read a few books on labour and delivery but found they frightened me, especially the books with great detail and graphic pictures.

My very dear friend Caroline lives in Nova Scotia in the summer and Northern Ireland for the rest of the year. She is a dancer and an artist and a storyteller. She suggested I talk to a friend of hers, Andrea, a nurse in Labour and Delivery at the hospital where we were going to have our baby. I called Andrea. She lives in a log cabin on the North Mountain. She is just five years older than me and has a grandchild. I would have loved to have had a home birth if I were a decade younger, but I didn't want to take any chances. Andrea said if we knew what we wanted, the hospital staff would work with us so we could have the kind of birthing we wanted. So we did up a detailed birth plan with Alice and reviewed it with our obstetrician, who signed a copy for us to hand in when we went to the hospital to deliver. It was all very tidy and organized, except for the great unknown of how to birth the baby.

I assumed labour would be short and fast. That was how I did things. Quickly. Intensely. I might be shy at first but would then jump right in like I'd been doing it all my life. That was how I did everything. Without hesitation. I would have the ideal natural childbirth — spiritual, calm, and controlled, no medication, no panic, no pain so big that I couldn't breathe my way through it.

THERE IS A PHOTO James took of me with the girls on our due date, October 23, 2005. It was just before supper, and we are standing near the barn in front of a sugar maple, the leaves cherry red against the blue sky. Looking at the photo I can remember how tired I was at that moment. I don't look tired, however. I look relaxed, happy, very young. I can remember so vividly the hours leading up to the labour. The girls are giggling in the photo. I was looking forward to going to bed as James took that picture. My back hurt more than it had for the entire pregnancy. I'd been plagued with back problems for the past several years, and I was surprised at how well my back had held up all the weight. I was wondering if it was a sign. I was looking for signs everywhere that last week, wondering if the baby would come early. Hoping, actually. I was worried I'd go beyond the due date and have to be induced. Some women had shared stories of being induced and how it quickly brought on a very hard and intense labour. This was my greatest concern as the day drew to a close with no baby — induction.

And there was so much to do after supper that night. Dishes to wash, clothes to fold, getting the girls to bed. James reading stories upstairs while I wondered how many days I would have before this child joined us. Me puttering about the house, watching James put another log on the fire as the evening became night. Standing to stretch my back. Standing outside in bare feet, looking up at the stars. I was so hot in those final weeks that the crisp October evenings were a balm on my roasting skin. There was a brilliant half-moon in the black night sky, the sky that sparkled as though handfuls of stars had been flung from the palm of a spinning child.

And I finally made it to bed at around 11:00 p.m. But my back kept aching, and I had a fitful hour of sleep. I felt like I had to pee and I finally got up and sat on the toilet. There was a bit of blood and I had a mild crampy feeling low in my abdomen. I went back to bed, but the cramp kept coming back.

I got up and called my friend Lynn, who was living in

Edmonton at the time. She'd had a baby years ago when she was a teenager. I was an old lady, but surely she could remember enough to tell me what was happening. I remember the floor cool on my feet as I walked downstairs to find the phone. I called her while I sat on the toilet.

"I'm having cramps," I said when she answered.

She replied, "Don't you mean contractions? It's not like you're on your period, you fool."

I said that perhaps I was in labour. She laughed and said she thought I might be, and that I should get off the phone with her and call the doula who lived on the North Mountain. Her last words were to be prophetic: "Remember, even if you have a long, hard labour, in the end it really isn't that much time, not for what you'll have when it's over."

But in the deep of the night, a baby was a lifetime away.

I called Alice at 3:00 a.m. No answer. I left a message. I had more cramps. *Contractions*, I reminded myself. I thought of a card I had received long ago. *She who hesitates is not only lost but miles from the next exit.* It wasn't a time to hesitate. *Contractions*, I repeated.

Alice called back. She wanted me to describe "the show." She wanted to know how much blood there was. I didn't know how to measure it. "More than before, when there was none," I said. Alice giggled and said she'd be there soon.

"Oh," she said, just before we ended the call, "how's James?"

"Oh," said I, "I don't know. He's still sleeping."

She giggled. "You better let him know."

And so I padded back upstairs and woke him up.

"Are you sure?" he asked.

"Yes," I said. "You sleep. Alice will be here. We'll get you up if we need you."

Alice arrived and examined my discharge. She said there wasn't actually that much blood, that I wasn't going to have the baby imminently. I remember she was shivering, so I made a fire for her while she lit candles and arranged them throughout the room, on windowsills, on tables and shelves, everywhere, until the space was filled with soft light and flickering shadows. She made me tea, raspberry leaf and nettle with maple syrup, as prescribed by my naturopath. She began to time my contractions, which were anywhere from eight to five minutes apart. I remember being exhilarated, feeling very alive, so thrilled that soon I would be holding my baby.

And here the memories blur. Alice writes in her story:

> *The early hours of Saturday, drinking tea in the quiet, creating a relaxing candlelit atmosphere to labour in, was most memorable, and I truly enjoyed our time while the girls and James slept. When Anna and Mary awoke early to see labouring Christy Ann and hear that the baby was on the way, they were very excited. They sat in their little pink armchairs by the fire with great anticipation for this baby they thought would just "pop out" at any moment. As the darkness of the night began to shift into day, the energy began to heighten; the peacefulness of the dark and quiet soon turned into the bustle of the day.*

Alice made me toast and encouraged me to eat. I wasn't hungry, but she assured me I would need the nourishment later. I was so excited I couldn't imagine feeling weak, but I did as she asked. Alice pointed out that I'd had only a few hours of sleep, and I'd need my energy. I thought she was being overly cautious. How long could all of this go on?

And I remember the house coming alive with James and the

girls, the calm and quiet booted out the door with the busyness of the morning household. I had to have quiet and peace — the chatter and noise and bustle were jarring. I wanted to be outside with the cool air and the morning sun.

Our friend Gwen arrived at 7:45 a.m., and she took charge of the girls so we could go for a walk. Alice hoped the walk would speed up my labour, which seemed to be stalling, with the contractions still coming anywhere between five and ten minutes apart. So we walked the Loop, a walk I'd done every day since I was seven months pregnant and my doctor had pointed out it was time to stop riding my bike through the woods before I fell off — it was a question of balance. The Loop is a wonderful walk on old-world country roads. You turn out of the farm and head up the South Mountain, and at the top you head east, looking down at the beautiful Annapolis Valley, the North Mountain, the endless sky stretching over the land. You then turn down into the valley for several more kilometres, finally looping back through the orchards to the cottage where we live, on a ninety-three-acre apple farm owned by lifetime friends, Waldo and Judy Walsh.

It's a spectacular walk, and here I've seen the seasons birth, grow, and pass in intricate detail. I know where the shadows fall depending on the time of day and time of year. I know the blackberry patches. I know there are eight bullet holes puncturing the metal slow sign on the side of the road coming down the mountain, holes shot by the yahoo who lives at the top of the mountain. I've seen the clouds cast galloping blue shadows over the valley's snow-covered fields. When we walked the Loop, the sky was blue and a white half-moon was high up in the eastern sky. A child's moon, Alice called it, the moon you can see in the daytime sky. I'd stop and bend over when I had a contraction. Alice kept timing me. I remember focusing very carefully on my belly and my back, still unsure if I was having a contraction. I hadn't expected them to be centred in my lower back, but at that point they were still manageable. When we were coming back through the orchard, Alice and James saw a Honeycrisp apple tree heavy with fruit, and they went bounding off through the orchard while I leaned against a large granite boulder at the side of the road. I remember the solitude of that moment, seeing the mountaintop as it brushed the brilliant blue sky. They ran back with arms full of apples. I remember laughing.

We arrived back at the house. The contractions hadn't progressed much in length or intensity, but I was beginning to feel very tired, so I went to bed. I was feeling anxious that things were going so slowly. It had been almost thirteen hours. My dear friend Marie called from California, and she told me how she had thought about sea anemones and jellyfish when she was in labour. She imagined herself riding big waves that would explode on the sand and then withdraw, only to flood back and break once more.

I can't remember more about the afternoon. The fatigue had begun to possess me.

James brought me blueberry pancakes and tea, and joined me in bed while Gwen took the girls off to gymnastics. I remember feeling the house settle, the quiet return, but still I could not sleep.

EARLY AFTERNOON. I AM UP. Alice suggests a hot shower and nipple stimulation to get the contractions going. It's been sixteen hours now that I've been in labour. The nipple stimulation is excruciating, and I can barely stand doing it, but it doesn't take long for the intensity of the contractions to increase dramatically. I can feel them in my lower back, and I have to get on my knees to handle the pain. It's late afternoon and I'm very tired and I want to go home. I am at home, of course.

The contractions are punctuated by Murray, the hired man, driving by on the tractor pulling great wooden bins of bright red apples to the tin shed. *There goes Murray* becomes the birthing mantra. We can time the contractions with his endless passings. None of this is what I'd expected. I feel so alone when I have a contraction. I can't stand any talk. We were playing music earlier, but I can't tolerate any noise now. I want only the sound of the wind in the autumn leaves, the crackling fire, whispers if there has to be talking. I feel as though I'm retreating from these people I love: James, who is tired and worried; Alice, who is always patient, rubbing my back and feeding me sips of tea and water. At some point Mary and Anna come home. They talk to me, oblivious to my pain. I bend over, unable to talk. Alice explains to them that the contractions are very strong now. They put their arms around me: *We know just how you feel*, they say. I remember smiling through the agony. They change and head off to play at Waldo and Judy's, and I won't see them again until the baby is born.

We continue labouring, now joined by Gwen, our dear friend from the Quaker meeting I am a member of. Gwen who is centred and calm, ready to do whatever is needed. She has never witnessed a birth, and graciously accepted our invitation to participate in the birthing. Her enormous laugh will ring out like a trumpet in the mists that are to surround me. She and Alice and I head off for another walk in the apple orchards, and the walk helps bring on longer and more intense contractions. The sky is now darkening with the end of day. I think of a friend who compared the endurance of birthing to the endurance of a marathoner. I have run a marathon, but it took only four hours to complete — a minor accomplishment compared to this. There seems no end in sight. I think of Lynn telling me that even if the labour is long, it really isn't.

Back inside they feed me orange juice and toast for supper. I know this only because I read it in Alice's story. At this point Alice calls a midwife she works with to consult her on the progress of my labour. She tells Alice to look for a purple line between my buttocks to get an idea of dilation. I kneel on the bathroom floor for Alice, who says the baby's about halfway up, about five centimetres, which means I'm approximately halfway dilated. Finally there is a shift in my labour. The contractions are long and painful and close together. Alice's notes say there were eight contractions in twenty-five minutes. I just remember I couldn't stand up anymore without James and Gwen holding me while Alice applied counterpressure to my lower back. It was the only way I could get through a contraction. I could only handle the contractions upright, but I was no longer able to stand, my runner's legs collapsing from bearing me and my mighty belly for eighteen hours.

Alice says that it's time to go to the hospital; it's time to leave the quiet, cozy cottage where the fire burns and the cats lounge. The sky hangs over us like a bruise—dark blue and red in the west, black in the east. Alice and I get in the car with James. Gwen follows in her car. I don't want the highway. I want to drive down Brooklyn Street, a country road that runs through the middle of the valley. I've forgotten that the road is also lined with bumps and potholes, and every one we hit is torture. I remember clinging to Alice, the pain almost unbearable. I want to stand but we are in a car. I cling to her like a child. It is dark outside. I cannot see stars. It is indeed a long way to Hectanooga.

I have a contraction outside the doors of the Valley Regional Hospital in Kentville, Nova Scotia, and then in the lobby. The idea of being enclosed in an elevator makes me sick. Someone comes at me with a wheelchair, and I run—or waddle—away.

We walk up the stairs to Labour and Delivery. I have a contraction at the top of the stairs.

At the hospital Andrea, the nurse who lives in the log home, is just finishing her shift. I feel like weeping when I see Andrea. I think of Caroline and her love of ritual and deep breathing. Andrea does my first internal—I am seven centimetres dilated and she can feel the bulge of my membranes. My water has not broken. Andrea leaves after assuring me that Carrie, who is coming on shift, will be wonderful. I trust Andrea completely. I remember Alice and Andrea talking. I am naked in the bathroom. They are in the doorway. Andrea says I'm entering transition. I think I'm entering hell. I remember from our labour classes with Alice that the contractions during transition are fast and intense, with little time in between: steep, steep mountains and tiny valleys. I remember she said the best thing about transition is that it rarely lasts an hour. Mine lasts for almost three. I am dripping with sweat, so hot, when having a contraction, and then shivering and so cold when it ends. I feel like vomiting and lean over the toilet, but I can't be sick. I want to pee and poop, but I can't do either. They cover me in a flannel sheet, and as soon as a contraction starts again I throw it on the floor. It now requires James, Alice, and Gwen to hold me upright, the only way I can stand the pain in my back.

They call my obstetrician, Dr. Singh. In rural Nova Scotia your baby is usually delivered by whoever is on call, but Dr. Singh has written on my chart that he is to be called. They reach him at a cocktail party, just, he says, after one drink.

I can't stand any touch on my flesh and refuse to wear a belt with a monitor. They ask if they can do periodic checks, and I agree. Once they insist on "doing a strip" to check the baby's heart rate. His heart rate is always fine. He is never in distress, not like his mother, who is in constant distress.

It is nighttime when they call Dr. Singh to come in and break my membranes. He has been in earlier: I remember seeing his white turban. He comes back. There is a great warm gush of water, and the release feels fabulous, but only for a few moments. The contractions continue to come at me like waves. I've always hated sailing, and I feel as though I'm trapped on a sailboat in a hurricane. Alice encourages me to keep with my breathing, but I can't remember how it goes.

"Long cleansing breaths," she's saying. "Short breaths, pants."

And it's then that I leave them. And it's there that my running days save me. Runners talk about hitting a wall — you cannot go on. But you run the race in your mind. You know you have to go through that wall. Beyond it lies renewal, rebirth. And so you continue, and then you are soaring. I cannot manage the pain anymore, so I retreat deep inside, where I am beyond my body, where I am beyond my mind, where I am in the heart of my being, where there is no doubt and hesitation, only pure light and dark. I can feel hands on me as the contraction starts, but I am no longer in the bathroom in our birthing room at the hospital. It is night and I am by a fire. My friend Caroline is there. It is a large bonfire surrounded by women, and the light of the flames casts us in gold. I feel the heat of the fire on my face, and I turn to Caroline, who is dancing. Sweat drips down my face and I lick my lips. The salt travels through my veins. Caroline reaches out her arms to me, gesturing to me to join them. She is moving from foot to foot in a slow, rhythmic march. She is chanting, and I let my breath join hers.

And then I am back in the hospital bathroom, shivering with a sheet around my shoulders. When the next contraction comes, I hear Caroline call me in her low voice and I return to the fire. She does not smile, just looks at me, chanting. And so it continues for the next two hours. When the contractions come, I know I must join Caroline or I cannot endure the pain. James and Gwen and Alice join this new breathing. I can hear them, though I cannot see or feel them anymore.

Finally I am too tired to stand, and lying down, the pain in my lower back is beyond endurance. I am seized with fear when a contraction comes and Alice is not there. I can no longer reach Caroline, not while lying down on this hospital bed. I am trapped in my body. I remember wanting the epidural then. I remember insisting. I remember the discussion, the reminders that I hadn't wanted one.

"Get me a fucking epidural," I say.

Someone, maybe Alice, says to Gwen that she just wants to make sure I really want one. Gwen says it seems clear to her that all I want is an epidural. And that is when they call Dr. Singh, who says it's too late. He says I can have laughing gas instead. I can't believe it. I hate him. The first gulp works. With the teeny bit of clarity I momentarily possess, I tell them I want to go home and sit by the fire with the cats. They laugh and say that I have to push the baby out if I want to do that. I want them all to die. I want to die.

AFTER THAT FIRST GULP, the laughing gas only makes me feel sick. It seems there is no relief. Somewhere in the midst of this pain and exhaustion I think of my Estonian theatre history professor at the University of Ottawa. I remember her talking about childbirth, how halfway through she'd had enough, that she was done. And she said she realized that there was no turning back; she just hadn't known this before. Then I think of Vsevolod Meyerhold, a theatre director, actor, and playwright in Russia following the revolution. He believed in a connection between body and emotion, the connection between the physiological and the psychological. He was a victim of the Stalinist purges. He was sent to a camp and shot. I think around then I have another contraction, and I forget about poor old Meyerhold.

Dr. Singh arrives at some point after the birthing crew has decided I am now ready to push. He is wearing a wool toque. He says I should push. He is obviously insane. I cannot push. I have to get out of this place, but there is no exit.

AND THEN THE CONTRACTIONS started. I know there was an early one and I refused to push I was so angry. And then the next one came and I refused to push, but somehow I was pushing. A voice in the room said, "Even if she won't do it, her body will do it for her."

I remember not understanding how to push. I could barely tell when I was having a contraction at this stage. I was shocked at not knowing something that should be instinctive. Another betrayal. It was like my body and I were separate now. It was going to push the baby out because I didn't know how to. I wasn't a willing participant. There was such enormous pressure from the waist down. I kept remembering the *ring of fire*. I didn't want the ring of fire, but it had found me.

Nurse Carrie sat beside me and put her fingers in my vagina. She asked if I could feel them, and I think I nodded.

"Push them out," she said.

I could do that. Everyone was so tired then except for Carrie. And then the baby's head crowned. A voice asked if I wanted to see the baby's head. I had packed a mirror, a gilded mirror, on the advice of my friend Lisa in Newfoundland. She said it would give me encouragement to see the baby's head. But when they asked if I wanted to see it, I recoiled. The idea of breaking my concentration was anathema. Dr. Singh told me to feel the baby's head. I reached down. It was warm and soft and squishy. *Oh my God*, I thought, *I'm going to poke my finger into his brain, and he'll be a vegetable.* I snatched my hand back. I think they laughed at this too.

And then Carrie was saying it was time to push the baby out. His head kept coming almost halfway out and then slipping back in. She told me I had to do three pushes on the next contraction—I had been managing only two. And she wanted me to bear down. I remembered from our birthing classes that bearing down was something you should avoid doing unless you were having trouble, unless you need some superhuman pushes. And so on that contraction I became superhuman and bore down and I gave Nurse Carrie the three pushes she wanted. Silas, all eight pounds, eleven ounces, came out. It was 2:54 a.m.

After his birth I remember only bits. They put the baby in my arms, but I was so weak he was slipping down my chest. My arms were numb. I couldn't smile at him. He latched on to my breast right away while those enormous dark eyes locked on to mine. I was in love. And Dr. Singh asked me to push again. I raised my head and looked at him. Just a little one, he said. And out came the placenta. He held it up and showed it to me. It was enormous and looked like a huge piece of meat. It was one of the biggest he'd ever seen, he said. He showed me how it would have been positioned in the uterus, how the cord attached to it. I wanted to ask him questions, but I was too weak, too foggy. And my arms were still so numb and the baby was slipping and then he was pooping all over me. They were cleaning us both up, and suddenly I was alive, surges of energy going through me like lightning. I had a baby. He was healthy. He was almost nine pounds. He had dark eyes and hair. I was starving. They served me toasted sourdough raisin bread and cheese and sparkling peach juice. I remember the drawn faces of the people in the room. James's face was so long, even with his smile, his hand on my forehead as he looked at me and Silas. I had gone into labour on Friday night and it was now Sunday morning. And they left me and went home to get some sleep while I held my beautiful baby, who smelled like the gardens of paradise.

IF I COULD DO IT again, would I have had pain medication earlier? Would I go to the hospital to be induced and skip the long labouring at home? I don't know. I believe my fear of being a mother, my worry about not being ready, my fear of the unknown slowed my labour. I kept thinking about all the things I wanted to do that I hadn't done yet. Would a baby keep me from doing them? Would I be able to accept the changes a child would bring? Would I be a resentful parent? I'm sure these thoughts had much to do with my age and my biology, but I know that my trepidation about being a parent came into direct conflict with my body. And the body always wins.

I didn't have the ideal labour, the quick and speedy labour I had anticipated. After I had Silas, what I realized is that I have, in fact, hesitated for much of my life. I had spent many years being miles from the next exit. I might have made decisions quickly but then I'd dither, become fearful, noncommittal. Since having Silas I do not hesitate, not like I once did. His birth, his life, my life with my family have given me a clarity and precision in living.

For some time after his birth, the memory remained immediate and visceral. The soreness, the tenderness, all testimony to the experience. It is something you recount again and again to those who ask, and to some who don't. There's a compulsion to share the story, especially with other women who have been through the experience of labour and birth. I say little to someone who is pregnant. There will be time when their baby has come. I believe that this storytelling, this sharing of birth stories, is a way of integrating the experience into your being, into memory. But somewhere along this road the memory starts to transform. It becomes a memory of a memory. I'm not sure exactly when, but for me it was sometime around the end of the first year. I remember thinking that I could never forget such a primitive ordeal. But as my body healed, and as my baby grew, the memory transformed. As I was told so often before I had my son, the reward for such a trial is so magnificent that it overshadows all. And this is true.

And now when I think back to the birthing, I find that, rather than a disruption or a distortion, there has been a seasoning and a softening of the memory — a patina has been painted over the recollection. And there is this tiny new voice that at first coos and gurgles and laughs and babbles, then utters a few words that fall into hilarious sentences. The baby who delights in his first independent splash of tub water; the toddler who notices a shadow and chases it, calls to it, perplexed by its aloofness; the tiny one who points up to the sky one dark autumn night and says, "Look, Mama, moon, up in the sky."

I am humbled that this being has brought me such exquisite joy and fear and courage. The pain of his birth is a memento from a long journey, like the leaves Alice collected as we looped through the countryside during labour, the leaves she placed on the cover of the birth story, which have now dried, their edges preserved in perfect detail but the colour and texture altered forever.

HELPLESS

Curtis Gillespie

PARIS MAY BE THE world's most romantic city, but it can also be a place like any other, a place where misfortune and contingency have a say, no matter how beautiful the backdrop. In mid-July of 1998 I found myself sitting on a hard wooden bench in the tenebrous light of a long, empty hallway in the Hôpital Val-de-Grâce in the 5th arrondissement. It was late morning. I was alone. I didn't know what to do. Twenty minutes earlier my poor French had prevented me from getting a proper report from the duty nurse, who did not speak English.

"Can you please tell me where my wife is?" I had asked her. "What's happening? Where's my wife?"

The nurse tried to smile, said something in French, stopped, switched to rudimentary English. "Please. Wait. Operation... under way." She motioned for me to sit.

"Operation?" I said. "What operation?"

She struggled for words in English, couldn't find them, motioned to the bench again. I sat. Operation? Where was my wife?

Where was the doctor, any doctor? The nurse said no more and walked away, leaving me to the bench, to my ignorance and fear.

We had gone to the hospital earlier that morning, four hours before, because Cathy suspected she'd had a miscarriage (and she had also had stiffness in her shoulders for about a week, which no amount of Aspirin or massage seemed to relieve). Her doctor back in Edmonton had said over the phone that once she was sure she'd miscarried, she needed to get to a hospital and get a RhoGAM shot because of her Rh blood type.

The waiting room at Val-de-Grâce was full, which was surprising because it wasn't even 8:00 a.m. We'd left our flat without eating breakfast, so I nipped out to the local *boulangerie* to pick up croissants and coffee while Cathy waited. We had a houseful of visitors that week, including my mother and grandmother, and our thinking in going so early was that we could be back in time to have a full day, given that it was the birthday of our three-year-old daughter, Jessica.

After finishing our coffee and croissants and sitting for another hour, Cathy and I agreed that I ought to head back to the flat to check up on everyone. Not that we were worried, but my granny wasn't exactly in the best of health; every day upon returning to our flat, she'd ascend the stairs to our third-floor walk-up, flop onto a kitchen chair, light a cigarette, and wheeze out, "Ginandtonic ... ginandtonic."

Cathy phoned about ten.

"It's just so busy here, and I'm still waiting," she said, clearly frustrated. "The last thing I want to do is sit around here all day." But leaving would only mean going through the wait again the next day; she needed the RhoGAM shot within seventy-two hours. She hung up. After yet another hour, I left our flat and walked back to Val-de-Grâce. It was closing in on noon by this time. Cathy wasn't in the waiting room when I got there. Assuming she was in with a doctor, I sat and waited for fifteen minutes before finally going up to the desk to try to ask how long ago it was that she'd gone in to talk to the doctor and get her needle. The clerk looked at me with some alarm, and then called for the duty nurse.

———

THREE YEARS EARLIER TO the day, we were also in a hospital, in Edmonton, where Cathy was giving birth to our first daughter. The pregnancy had gone as smoothly as one could hope, and perhaps that's why one of the overriding memories of the birth of our first daughter was that it was all more or less under control. Cathy was on top of it and didn't seem nervous, so I wasn't either. However, a week or so after the due date, the baby hadn't given many signs of wanting out, so our doctor decided Cathy needed to be induced. After a few hours at the hospital, the pain began to roll in on waves, but it was too late by then for an epidural. She got some morphine, which blunted the pain but also made her a bit dopey, caught in that netherworld of drowsy yet severe discomfort. We spent a lot of time walking up and down the hallways, trying to keep moving, stay awake, waiting for the contractions to increase.

When it finally did happen I was an absolute mess, bawling my eyes out for most of it (though this may have been due to Cathy's squeezing my hand like a dishrag—a warning to men soon to be in the same position: take off your wedding ring to avoid crushed fingers). When the head appeared, Cathy was pushing, pushing, pushing, pushing, pushing, groaning, half-yelling;

the doctors, the nurses, me, all urging her to push some more, that she was nearly there, that she was doing such an amazing job, that she was nearly there, that she *was* there, that *we saw something*, and then suddenly, in a spilling, bloody, glorious rush, our child surged out, as if she (though we didn't yet know she was a she) simply couldn't wait another second to come into the world. The head appeared first, up to the neck, and the next surge brought the rest of her out. I told Jessica recently that we met her before we even knew she was a girl. "That's weird," she said, thinking about it for a minute. "Kind of gross."

I thought it ironic then, and still do, that in the birth room the one person doing all the work, taking all the risk, feeling all the pain, is the person with the worst view of the proceedings. I wondered if women ever felt a bit ripped off at having the worst seat in the house, as it were. But despite having the best seat in the house, I am quite certain I was more messed up than anyone present. Being the relevant man at a birth is a peculiar position to be in, because you feel—or at least I felt—at once deeply central to what is going on but also entirely peripheral. This feeling seems inescapable to me, no matter what your partner tells you (as in "You were such a big help"; "You were there and I felt you were there, and it meant a lot"; "I couldn't have gone through it without you there"—all of which Cathy told me). Despite all these expressions of appreciation and partnership (that part of me thinks are what women say only because they are smart enough and forgiving enough to know that men, even when something is patently not about them, still want to think it is about them), despite all these things your partner will tell you, and despite the fact that this living creature about to enter the world is partly yours, despite all of this, deep, deep down men know that during the delivery they are just baggage. Not bad baggage or painful baggage (one hopes), but baggage all the same. Men get it. They know the truth: someone else, someone stronger and braver and tougher and more resilient than they will ever be, is carrying the whole can in that room.

Men are just hangers-on, basically, delivery-room roadies, because a man (or at least this man) knows as he witnesses this staggeringly emotional event that it's all going to go ahead whether he is there or not, whether he is supportive or not, whether or not he displays his caring and sensitivity and massage skills and icechip skills and supportive skills. That baby is coming out of that woman, now, today, and nothing's changing that. Witnessing the birth of my first child made me feel more helpless than I have ever felt in my life. Not useless, I don't mean that. But helpless. The agony of that level of helplessness is enough to make you want to jump off a bridge or throw yourself under a car, so heavy is the weight of your inability to make things better or speed the course of events or ameliorate the pain of this person you love.

My wife was in the strangling grip of a harsh and beautiful biological struggle, as is every woman who delivers a child, but all I could do was rub her back, hold her hand, tell her how great she was. It sure didn't feel like much. Bearing witness to it was miraculous, but humbling. If you witness your partner, your love, go through this and you don't fall in love with that person again to a new depth of your heart and being, then you weren't paying attention. This is an essay about the birth of my children, but it's really only partly about that, because during those moments when my children were in the very midst of entering this world, I wasn't really thinking about them much at all. I was thinking about my wife. In such moments, when someone you love is in pain, for whatever reason, your love and worry are largely defined by your feelings of helpless awe.

After Jessica emerged into the world, the placenta wouldn't dislodge from the uterus, so Cathy, without much time to enjoy her newborn, had to go into surgery under general anesthetic. She came through it with no complications but needed another few days in the hospital. We finally returned home one fine July morning and got all settled, at which point a ferocious noise began shrieking away in our front yard. We had a dead birch in the yard, and Cathy's sister and a friend had chosen that day, of all days, to come over and spend five or six hours hacking up the tree, their two chainsaws roaring away not twenty feet from the bedroom where Cathy was trying to recover. In retrospect it seems an apt metaphor for the noise and excitement and activity that is child-rearing; peace and quiet are not factors in a house with children—at least not our house. There's always a figurative chainsaw of one sort or another roaring away in family life, and occasionally a real one too.

———

THE SILENCE IN THE Val-de-Grâce hallway was shattered by the double set of swinging doors bursting open, just the way they always do on *ER*, the gurney wielded like some medieval battering ram. I looked up. It had been an hour since anyone had spoken to me, and there had been nothing to do but wait. Two attendants were pushing the gurney, not frantically, but with purpose. A doctor and a nurse were trailing in its wake, surgery gowns flapping like manta wings. I looked up as the gurney passed a few feet from where I sat. A spear of recognition and fear went through the middle of me.

"That's my wife!" I shot up off the chair. "That's Cathy! That's my wife. What's going on? What was the operation for?"

The doctor stopped. He didn't smile, though that wasn't so unusual in Paris. The gurney with Cathy on it kept moving, propelled by the two orderlies and the nurse. They turned a corner at the end of the hallway and disappeared. I wanted to run after them, but the doctor didn't seem to want to follow. He considered me briefly and then decided to smile, which nearly brought me to tears.

"It was a very serious situation," he said in passable English. "She did not miscarry at all. Her pregnancy was ectopic."

He told me that Cathy had been very, very fortunate. The ectopic fetus had ruptured her Fallopian tube, probably many days earlier. The hemorrhaging had been so severe that her sore shoulders were not the result of stiffness but of massive internal bleeding creating pressure on her thorax and upper body. The doctor said he had removed many pints of blood and blood clots, and that Cathy had literally been within hours of "falling into a coma and quite possibly dying." I thought back to the brief discussion we'd had earlier that morning about her wanting to leave the hospital. If she hadn't needed the RhoGAM shot (which, as it turned out, she actually didn't need), she'd have left and might now have been in, or well on her way to, a coma.

I sat on the bench for a moment, and then we went together into the room where Cathy's bed was now anchored. She was still unconscious, a needle drip in her arm. The doctor continued, explaining that when he met with Cathy earlier that morning, she'd said she'd had a miscarriage. He did some blood work, the results of which gave him pause and made him think that it wasn't a miscarriage. A laparoscopy was required to rule out an ectopic pregnancy. Cathy had had to sign a consent form allowing him to operate immediately in the event that the laparoscopy indicated a need. There had been some language confusion as to exactly what she was signing, but she signed in the end.

What it all really meant was that this was a very thorough doctor who hadn't simply accepted that Cathy had had a miscarriage, given her a shot of RhoGAM, and sent her on her way. He wanted to double-check. That double-check might have saved her life.

"Thank you," I said to him, looking over at Cathy. "Thank you so much."

He nodded and said, "Not a problem," as if it was something he did every day, which maybe he did, I don't know. After he left, I found a phone and called the flat, explained to my mum what had happened, and then got Jess on the phone to wish her a happy birthday from her mum, and that I'd be home soon to pick her up so we could visit her mum together in the hospital.

———

I WOULD NEVER SAY THAT having our first child was *easy*, because that's not something I'm in a position to declare. But what I can say about having Jessica is that I expected it to be profoundly moving, I expected that it would be hard and painful for Cathy, I expected that I would not know exactly what to do or how to help or where to stand. I expected to be filled with love for our new child, and for my wife. In all these things my expectations were more or less fulfilled. It was all exciting and new, but it still fell within the parameters of what I had been anticipating.

But in Paris I saw much more deeply into the possibilities of what childbirth is, into what it is women go through each time this process begins. Having a baby is hardly the peril it once was (at least not in the industrialized world), and it remains a moving and meaningful thing, but it is also, simply, a risky business.

My wife was close to dying because we wanted to have another child. I'd not included this within the boundaries of all the things that could happen.

Trying again after Paris was fraught with more than the usual complications. In the operation Cathy had had one tube removed. Neither of us was getting any younger. We never really did talk about not trying again; it just seemed apparent to both of us that it was the thing to do. And once we were back living in Edmonton, Cathy did indeed get pregnant again and carry to term.

It went smoothly, and in most ways, Cathy has said, it was an easier pregnancy and delivery than with Jessica. When it was over, that same sense of helplessness flooded out of me and was replaced with love and relief and something else that I can only describe as a kind of awe towards what my wife was capable of, an awe at how miraculous one single birth is and yet how regularly it actually happens. Soon enough Cathy was holding our newborn. She was exhausted, naturally, but blissed out too. Jessica was there with us. We didn't say much. Just rested together, a family.

"I have a name," Cathy said, looking up to me from our new child. We had talked a bit about names to that point, but hadn't settled on anything.

I looked back at her. She said the name. I smiled. It was perfect, of course. It was the only possible name, and said everything that needed saying, said everything we were feeling. I can't say for certain we were conscious of it at that moment, but it was a name that said so much about the why and where, about what had been lost and gained. Maybe it was only later that we understood.

"Hello," whispered Cathy to the quiet new life in her arms, saying our new daughter's name for the first time. "Hello, Grace."

THE SPACES IN BETWEEN

Jaclyn Moriarty

I.

Lily, 1943
I was living in a flat at the top of Auntie Lou's house. The arrangement was that, when the baby started coming, Auntie Lou would run up to Mr. White's shop and Mr. White would telephone a taxi.

So that's what happened. The taxi came and took me to the hospital.

It was the Mater Hospital in North Sydney.

The steps up to Maternity were covered in frost.

Diane, 1968
I was at the evening college sewing class making a pretty pink dress when my water started leaking. So I suggested to my friend Dorothy that we go home a little early that night. After I dropped Dorothy off, I had a pretty strong contraction, which did worry me a bit. So when I got home, I ran inside and said to Bernie, "We had better go to the hospital."

We had never been to the hospital before and didn't know where to go when we arrived. We could see a Maternity sign but no driveway to get there. So Bernie drove down a flight of steps.

Jaci, 2006

I bought a pecan pie and a chocolate hedgehog and took them to my friend Sarah's place for afternoon tea.

Sarah's chairs were extremely uncomfortable. They hurt my lower back. I moved quietly to the couch. The couch was angled in such a way that it caused intense lower back pain. I slipped down to the floor but it was too late: the furniture had ruined my back.

I tried doing yoga stretches, but they only worked for three minutes at a time, then two minutes, then one.

After a while Sarah remembered how contractions work. I phoned Colin on his cell.

We drove to the Mater Hospital in North Sydney and took the lift up to Maternity.

⌣

2.

Lily, 1943

Well, I had been pretty sick with the pregnancy.

Viv was training with the air force down in Melbourne, so I'd been down there to live with him for a while. Oh, I went down in style. In a DC-3 plane, a beautiful plane. They weighed you first, on big scales, with your suitcase, then they took you by coach to the airport.

We stayed in a lovely room with a Mrs. Peel. In her big house.

Diane, 1968

I can't remember getting morning sickness, but I had to run out of the kitchen whenever I cooked lamb chops.

I remember Doctor Love saying, *Don't eat the fresh bread every day when the baker comes.* Because otherwise you'd gain too much weight. I can't remember any other rules.

The nurses were all in love with Doctor Love.

There was a class at the hospital run by a nurse. She was tall and had an angular face, and she was all dressed up in her uniform, with a veil. She told us to sit on the floor with our legs crossed when we watched TV. Because that would stretch your cervix. And babies need booties. And buy clothes in size two. Because they grow, you know. And don't let them rule your lives.

Jaci, 2006

I spent most of the pregnancy Googling cures for morning sickness. I was not allowed to eat soft cheese, processed meat, premade salad, pâté, sushi, shellfish, swordfish, smoked salmon, smoked trout, or king mackerel. Also: no lakes, no hot tubs, no hot baths, and no cleaning out the cat litter. If you do not drink at least four glasses of milk a day, said the *New York Post*, it is an insult to your unborn child.

At the prenatal classes we were told to pack a bag specifically for labour, including a printout of our birth plan, aromatherapy oils, a tennis ball for back massage, a wheat pack, favourite CDs, and candies to keep our Support Person awake. They showed us a video on the benefits of epidural anesthesia. We were split into groups to discuss Pain Relief and given sheets of butcher paper. Our group had to list the advantages and disadvantages of nitrous oxide and pethidine.

Lily, 1943
After five months I was pretty sick with the pregnancy, so I came back home to Sydney.

But the war had gotten worse; the Japanese had taken over Singapore then. You couldn't cross state borders. You needed a permit. I had to take a train home, and even then it was a troop train.

Diane, 1968
In the last weeks of the pregnancy I did a sewing course so I could make baby clothes. I remember I cleaned the house. I sure cleaned that house a lot. Stupid house. Bernie was doing shift work then, and I was always carrying in loads of wood to keep the fire going.

Jaci, 2006
I was seven months pregnant when Colin went to Canada on a business trip.

"Don't forget to ask your partner for a back rub!" advised www.babycentre.com.

"But he's in Canada!" I said, deeply concerned.

He emailed every day. *"I love you so much,"* he wrote. *"That so is the noise in the mind of an eagle leaping off a cliff and pumping its wings in delight."* He sent messages specifically for Baby: *"Please tell Baby there are such things as seeds that blow in the air from cottonweed trees; warm summer nights; pizza."*

I planned a holiday on the coast for when he returned. A month before the baby, we sat on the terrace of an ocean-view room and studied the "Pamper Me!" brochure for massage and manicure options.

Lily, 1943

And then, after the baby was born, we were not allowed out of bed for twelve days. Our feet were not allowed to touch the ground. Oh, we were very well cared for. The nurses gave us sponge baths: they would bring hot, steaming water in steel jugs. And they brought the baby to be fed, but otherwise you were left to rest.

The care and food were out of this world. Such good attention! It was like a holiday. For a lot of women it was the only holiday they ever got.

The wards were so sterile and sparkling. I was in a room for four people and I met the nicest folk. One girl had a husband who was an officer in the army, and she had two older boys, but her boys, of course, were not allowed in the hospital. She would wave to them from our window. Another girl knew of a cousin of mine who had got a chill the year before and died.

Diane, 1968

You stayed in for a week. The babies were in the nursery, of course. I was in a ward of eight ladies, one of whom had twins. I was jealous of her! Another lady had had a baby boy, and we decided to become friends. Her name was Shirley, and we still send a letter with a Christmas card to this day.   ·

Jaci, 2006

I was allowed to stay for three days. "We encourage you to get dressed," the nurses said repeatedly. "Get dressed as soon as possible! Walk around! Go to classes! This is not an illness!"

There was a white control panel with buttons for adjusting the angle of the bed or switching on the TV (which cycled through baby-care information programs).

Lily, 1943
The nuns all wore their habits. We had the kindest American
nun, all dressed in a white habit. Her name was Sister Patrick,
and she taught the new mothers how to breastfeed. She came in
of a morning and arranged flowers on a table in the centre of the
ward. We always had daffodils and Geraldton wax.

Diane, 1968
In those days they were very particular about chest X-rays for
TB, and the nurses would come around and announce that we
all had to go down to X-ray. I, of course, did what I was told, but
I did mention to the nurse that my breasts were swollen, and
so sore that someone had just wrapped them in a huge piece
of material with a whole lot of safety pins to keep it in place. It
was wonderful how the pain had disappeared. The nurse said
it didn't matter!

Off I went with some other women—it was a very long walk
and I felt sick. When we got there the people said take everything
off, and I took ages undoing all the safety pins. All the other ladies
finished way before me. As soon as I got the pins undone the pain
came back and I was crying, but the X-ray people just ignored
me. I couldn't wrap it back properly by myself and was very, very
unhappy. I vowed next time I would say no, but guess what, there
never was a next time, because the government decided we didn't
need chest X-rays anymore!

Jaci, 2006
Each day a different midwife introduced herself. "Hello! My
name's Jeannie, and I'll be taking care of you today!" There were
classes to teach you how to wrap the baby ("like a burrito!" the
husbands joked) and how to recognize Tired Signs. There was a

clipboard by the bed with a form to fill in each time you breastfed: *left side, 20 mins, sucked very well.* A lactation consultant arrived with an electric pump.

Lily, 1943
Now of course, the year before this, we'd just moved in to the flat at Auntie Lou's house. It overlooked the harbour. And one Sunday night I came home and there was Auntie Lou playing dominoes and eating candies with her brother and Mr. White. That's what they did on a Sunday.

So anyhow, we heard this dreadful booming noise.

And Uncle Fred said, "Don't worry, they're only doing the blasting for the Captain Cook Dry Dock."

Well, the next morning I went up to the Chinese grocer's and he said, "Did you hear the Japanese bombing the harbour last night?" And do you know, they'd followed a warship in through the boom gates — three small Japanese submarines had got through the gates into the harbour — and that's what the booming noise had been.

Diane, 1968
One day while I was still at the hospital, I was walking along the corridor (on the second floor) to go to the bathroom. I stopped to talk to another lady from our ward, and as we chatted we heard a strange roaring sound and the building started to rock. We were standing outside a boiler room, and we agreed that the boiler might blow up. We also agreed that we shouldn't be there when it did! So she went back to the ward and I carried on to the bathroom, quite fascinated that the floor was going up and down under my feet! I said to myself, "The wind sure rocks this old building."

When I came happily back from the bathroom, I was amazed to find pandemonium in the ward. Ladies were crying, nurses were rushing around putting everyone in bed, and Shirley was being marched along with her baby in her arms. You were not allowed to carry your baby; you always had to push it in its bassinette. I thought to myself, *I wonder what's wrong with Shirley.*

The nurses pulled the blinds down at the windows and said we had to have a rest.

After a while the matron came around (a very big deal) and was introduced to each of us by a nurse. When she came to me, the nurse said, "This is the calmest mother in the ward." I was very proud.

I did not say a word about the fact that I hadn't known it was an earthquake. (Apparently Shirley had grabbed her baby and was going to run out of the building!)

Jaci, 2006

The first night, I shared a room with a woman who was pregnant with twins. She had complications, she told me, and was supposed to rest. Then she set to work running her cattle farm by phone.

That same day a midwife took my blood pressure. She was an older woman, maybe in her sixties. "I wonder if you've noticed my fingernails," she said. I had noticed them. The tip of each was carrot orange. "It's henna," she said. "I got it in Morocco. Didn't know you couldn't get it off. It's finally growing out now." I liked her, so I asked about postnatal depression. "Is there something troubling you?" she asked. Behind the curtain, the twins lady grew still.

Lily, 1943

They hadn't got the big American ship, the *Chicago*, but they'd blasted the *Kuttabul*, a training ship in the harbour, and killed all the young boys training.

Two of the Japanese submarines blew themselves up, but they didn't know what happened to the third. It disappeared.

So anyhow, the next Sunday night we were all in bed asleep, and there's that blasting again! I was terrified. The week before I hadn't known what it was, of course, so I wasn't frightened. But when I knew, I did feel bad. We went under the stairwell and I made a cup of tea for Uncle Fred. Auntie Lou was deaf, so she stayed in bed.

Diane, 1968

It was a public holiday when the earthquake happened, so there were not many people in the city and nobody was hurt. A church steeple fell down. And the country town of Meckering (where the epicentre was) was flattened I believe.

For the next few days there were aftershocks, and all the windows in the hospital would rattle. Plus, when I was at home, sitting on the bed to feed the baby, the mirror on the dressing table would sway back and forth.

I was just as scared then as all the other mothers!

Jaci, 2006

A few days after the baby was born, divers discovered the lost submarine, the third submarine that had come into Sydney Harbour during the Second World War.

Lily, 1943

After I left the hospital, I went to stay at my mother's place because Viv was away at the war.

They sent him to Borneo and Malaysia, and he finished up at Morotai.

I didn't miss him because I had the baby. That sounds dreadful, doesn't it, not missing him, but we were all in the same boat. All my friends had babies and husbands who were away at war, and we'd get together at each other's houses and have lunch. Or we'd go to the cinema.

My mother was a dressmaker, and she worked in a big sewing room in our house. Her customers would come in and the baby would be asleep on the verandah, and they'd all peep in at her. She was a bit spoilt. Oh, she was a good baby. So long as you pushed the pram back and forth, she'd go to sleep.

We used to make cakes to send to the soldiers and put them in round tins with lids. We'd sew them into calico bags and send them to Malaysia and Borneo.

So, you know, we all kept very busy.

You had ration books then, of course, for your butter and sugar and flour. But the people next door had a cow. So they'd give us milk and cream.

And when Viv came back, he looked so thin and yellow! I hardly knew him myself, and the baby certainly didn't know him. She was two and half years old by then, and she didn't like him at all. But he soon got around her.

Diane, 1968

For most of that year Bernie was away up north, doing survey work for the iron ore mining on Mount Tom Price.

Joan next door was lovely. I remember one day I went running into her place crying and I said, "The baby's awake and I haven't even had my breakfast!" So she took the baby and bathed her for me.

Another time, a lady I knew was in town on holiday and she said, "Come out with us for the day." Well, I said no because I thought I couldn't possibly go out for a day. It just seemed too hard. And then I spent all day crying because I really did want to go.

And Shirley and I used to visit each other, even though she lived way across the city. I would catch the bus to her place, and the big old pram was put on hooks on the back of the bus. I wonder why the mattress and sheets didn't fall out as it sailed along. It was worth the trip, because Shirley cooked the most delicious sponge cakes.

Jaci, 2006

Colin flew back to Canada when the baby was four weeks old. I saw him off at the front door, smiling wide-eyed at the taxi driver, and did not cry.

My mother came around with a frozen lamb casserole. My grandmother sent a card with a kind message and a twenty-dollar note taped inside. My sister came by with salmon, coriander, mint, and couscous and made dinner while I fed the baby. We had chocolate ice cream for dessert and watched the season finale of ER.

Another sister visited and we took our babies for walks in their prams. A young man approached carrying a chainsaw. "Haircuts for the babies?" he said. "On special today!"

"No thanks," my sister said smartly, walking her three-wheeler pram.

—

3.

Lily, 1943
So that's what happened. The taxi came and took me to the hospital.

It was the Mater Hospital in North Sydney.

The steps up to Maternity were covered in frost. Had a darling baby.

Diane, 1968
We could see a Maternity sign but no driveway to get there. So Bernie drove down a flight of steps.

A nurse told me it was hospital procedure that everyone have a pethidine injection when they first arrived. I said that I had not heard about that before, but she repeated that it was hospital procedure, and me being the dutiful person who always does as she is told, I said no more!

I went sound asleep and woke up to find people all around me, including my doctor and a nurse telling me not to push yet. I didn't even know I was. I must have been doing it in my sleep. They said, "Now you can push," and I, of course, dutifully did, but I wondered to myself, *Do they know how much this hurts?*

Then I had a lovely sensation of a warm, rubbery hot water bottle sliding out of me, and there was Jaci. Her little face was all red, so I turned to the nurse and said, "Don't worry, they grow more beautiful." She quickly put me in my place as she snapped, "They are never so beautiful as the day they are born!"

Jaci, 2006

We drove to the Mater Hospital in North Sydney and took the lift up to Maternity.

"The first thing we suggest," said the midwife, "is that you take a bath."

I tried to think about the nature of contractions. Maybe a lid being tightened on a jar. Or the rotation of the gas cap on a car—that clicking noise it makes when you turn it in the wrong direction.

"Wait," I said, "I have to brush my teeth." The spaces in between were growing smaller. There was time to get my toothbrush but no time for the toothpaste. As each contraction surfaced, I ran across the room and clung to the side of an armchair. As it eased, I crept back to the basin. After five contractions my teeth were finally clean.

Colin filled the sunken bath, and I grew stern with the midwife. "This is wrong," I told her. "It's all in my lower back. If it moved to the front, I'd be okay." The midwife gazed at me. "Take a bath," she said, and walked out of the room.

But first I had to brush my teeth again.

In the bath I stared in wonder at my arms and legs. They were thin. I loved them in a way that was familiar: the way I'd loved my body when I was ten years old. In the last month of the pregnancy I'd eaten almost nothing and walked for hours each day. So my arms and legs were slender, but my belly was a crazy balloon. I watched the belly for tremors now, or surface undulations, but I guess the baby was busy being born.

I thought about the nature of contractions. An accordion, I thought. Or someone starting up a pull-string lawn mower. It's a sort of creaking turn. Or the vibrations of a chainsaw. It's—

The midwife was back. She was pursing her lips at me down in the bath.

"The contractions are still in the wrong place," I complained. "Are they?" she said rhetorically. Then she turned to Colin. "How high would you say her pain threshold is?" While Colin considered the question, the midwife drifted from the room.

I thought of a children's story I'd written the year before, about a girl who tries to stay dry in a storm by walking in the spaces between the raindrops. This was just as stupid. I was trying to get out of a bath and find a towel and dress myself and tidy my hair and brush my teeth again, all in the spaces in between.

Mind the gap, I thought. That made me laugh. *There is no gap! Ha ha!*

The midwife suggested foolish things. "Try straddling this!" She offered a big green ball. *You have no idea*, I thought, stridently, *just how much this hurts*. When she left the room I tried it once, then kicked the ball away.

"How about some gas?" she suggested when she returned.

"It doesn't help at all." I flew back to my armchair.

In the spaces in between I thought about contractions. It's a steering wheel, I thought, it's a ship's steering wheel that—turns until it catches, then turns and turns beyond—turns beyond the catch. There's a captain with powerful forearms turning the wheel so that—the captain turns the wheel beyond the catch so that machinery, levers, iron bars are slowly—it's a slow, majestic grinding, I thought, and machinery is slowly—slowly being splintered, no, cracked, then splintered, but—but despite the sounds of cracking, despite the crashing from the engine room, still the—the crashing from the engine room, the whole engine room, the ship, the whole—despite that, still the forearms—

I found I was on the bed. As long as I could reach for the gas mask—and then, when I was sure that it was gone, I'd hand the gas mask back. But sometimes the mask seemed to take my face with it.

I could only speak in single words, like this:

Where
Is
The
Baby?

Over and over I said it: "Where Is The Baby?" and Colin and the midwife laughed. They thought I was making a joke.

A new midwife had started her shift. She had my name wrong.

Her voice would approach from somewhere remote and say, "Okay, Jocelyn, how are you doing?" and each time I would plan a response:

Please
Don't
Call
Me—
That Is
Not
My—
I Am
Okay,
Thanks For Asking,
But, Listen
My
Name—

But before I had my reply ready, I'd have to grab the gas mask again.

"Focus on the rattling noise, Jocelyn!" the midwife said. "Make it rattle, that's a girl! Focus on that!" The rattle of the gas mask took me sideways for a moment.

"Where Is The Baby?" I said again, but I did not mean it as a joke. I meant, How could a baby survive this? Haven't we forgotten the baby?

"The baby's posterior," the midwife told me. "It's facing your back." Well, of *course*, I thought, I've been trying to tell you that for hours now.

It didn't matter anymore that the epicentre was my back. This was everywhere. This was lunging for the gas mask, gouging gasps of air, and digging fingernails into my arm. Once Colin tried to stop me, transferring my fingernails to his arm instead. I pushed him away in fury and returned to my own.

I wanted to say,

Is
Anybody—
or,
Does
Anybody
Know—

I wanted to say,

But
Why?

I thought about the nature of contrac—

I tried to think of —

Someone had taken a razor blade to my back. Sliced it horizontally, then slowly peeled the skin down to my feet.

No.

Someone had dismantled my body: the bones, the cartilage, the veins. Next they had affixed three plastic hooks, one in the centre of my back and one in each of my heels, and taken some freshly chewed gum, twelve or fifteen sticks of it, I think, and used this to rebind the body. The gum was now looped between the hooks. Somebody had gathered up the strings of gum, attached them to the bumper of a car, and driven the car to South Australia.

Afterwards Colin said, "That must be the loneliest place in the world — up on that bed in the labour ward." I agreed. It's the people speaking in everyday voices, making small jokes across the bed as if the space of the bed were surmountable, when you alone know that it is not. But then I thought, *No, there are lonelier places than that.*

"Right, Jocelyn," the midwife said. "I've spoken to your doctor on the phone, and he thinks that you need an epidural. He thinks otherwise you won't have the energy to push, and this will end up a Caesarean, okay?"

While she spoke, I thought about her voice. It had that tremble quality that some voices have, and this was the precise quality of the pain. I felt myself quiet as I heard each word, and her words were as separate as mine, only faster.

She was waiting for my response.

I tried to formulate one: *You see,* I formulated, *you see.*

It's not possible for me to have an epidural. What you don't understand is that a month ago, while we stayed in the ocean-view room on the coast, just after leafing through the "Pamper

Me!" brochure, Colin said he wanted to leave. While in Canada on his business trip, he said, he'd met somebody else. He wanted to fly back to Canada to be with her. He would try, he said, to stay, but couldn't promise.

Friends, when I told them, almost laughed. "That's just midsummer madness," said one. "*Everybody* knows that he loves you." Wait until he sees you giving birth, people promised. Over and over again. That puts everything in focus. This is a glitch, a temporary madness—but when he sees you giving birth, *that* will bring him back to himself.

So you see, this birth, this labour, has got to be perfect. I am drawing on the ancient mystical power of women, all women, giving birth. There can be nothing as modern or distorting as an epidural!

Also there is this: I am now in a world of gathering and gas mask. And once I saw a shadow on the ceiling that looked just like a tiny baby's profile. Here, in this world, is where I live now. This is where I'm safe. There are lonelier places than this: you could be in your own bed the night before last, the earliest cringes of contractions in your back, the front door quietly clicking, and there he is in his corduroy jacket, a whisky in his hand, heading to the pay phone up the road.

So leave me here in this alternate madness. Why interrupt with talk of epidurals? Why do you want to intrude?

But I could hardly speak at all, and that was seven paragraphs. How could I say all that in my separated words in the spaces in between? I was silent.

"Your doctor thinks you need an epidural," the midwife said again. "It's been seventeen hours already and he thinks that otherwise..."

She talked while I tried to summarize my paragraphs into a

single sentence. It would be something like *I Do Not Want An* —
I Am Okay, Thanks All The Same, But I Do Not —

"Where Is The Baby?" I said instead, and this time I said it to
remind myself.

"Jocelyn?" said the midwife.

"Okay."

I never saw the anesthetist's face. I was looking at the wall.
His voice seemed young and friendly, like a tennis player, eyes
alive with fun.

"You have to stay *perfectly* still," he said in his mischievous voice.
That was absurd. Did he not know you have to flee from it?
Contractions come in waves. That made me laugh. Contractions,
like grief and shock, come in monstrosities.

I stayed perfectly still and the room plunged into something
like pure, desperate suspense. I felt a jab and then the low-mur-
mured clutter of mistake. Something had gone wrong with the
needle. The medicine had splashed onto the floor.

A second time the anesthetist said, "You have to stay perfectly
still."

And behind me another jab, and this time even greater still-
ness, and then the friendly voice changed into something strange
and low. From far away I heard, "I've hit a blood vessel."

I wonder what that means, I thought, and then, more urgently,
Does that mean I'm going to die?

There was more busy movement.

And then, a third time, the anesthetist said, "Stay perfectly
still." But just as he said this, I screamed.

The scream was beautiful. A beautiful plummet. It was the
perfect manifestation of everything mad. In the world of this
scream I didn't have to brush my teeth or fix my hair or look
my best or make sense or be strong, but there was *strength*

in the scream, there was beautiful strength and surrender.

It was also the continuation of an earlier scream, the scream in the ocean-view room, a light, white room with nautical theme, cane chairs, and sunshine-striped carpet. That scream had followed hours of calm disentangling, figuring, figuring, figuring, *If I just say the right thing, there must be a way around, I'm going to make this make sense.* A dolphin turned like a graceful wheel and I screamed with a beautiful plummet, a plummet of surrender and defiance: the guests in the room next door.

"Okay, you ready?" the anesthetist said. "Stay perfectly—" But the midwife interrupted. "Wait! The baby's crowning! He's turned around!"

There were festive noises now, and the anesthetist was a tennis player again. A good sport who had just lost a friendly game. "I guess I won't be needed after all."

At last I spoke. In a strident voice, I said,

I

Do

Not

Need

An

Epidural.

There was quiet for a moment, and then they returned to their festivities.

The anesthetist left and the obstetrician arrived. He was wearing his weekend clothes.

"When you push," he said, "you'll feel like the world's being ripped apart."

Then he said, "I'll just get myself a cup of tea."

The pushing consisted of a lot of fanfare. Shouting and cheering, and I think someone was jumping up and down like a gorilla, but maybe I imagined that. The doctor gave elaborate, complex instructions. And he kept disappearing to get himself some chamomile tea. "By the time I get back," he'd say, "it'll all be over!" *Then why are you going?* I thought sternly. But it was always a lie. He'd return and things would still be underway. "You're pushing with your face," he told me once. He made no sense.

Some time later they plucked a baby from the table and placed him on my belly.

He was all floppy, slippery, dangling limbs like an octopus or a squid.

I really think I'm not being biased, I said to myself. *I really think I'm seeing clearly here. This baby is absolutely perfect!* I felt oddly panicked about this, as if someone should be notified.

———

4.

Jaci, 2006
The day after the baby was born, my grandmother arrived at the hospital with a bunch of sweet peas. "When I was here," she said. "I remember when I was here."

Lily, 1943
I remember when I was here, and after eight hours, or whatever it was, well, I fell asleep. And they woke me up, a nurse woke me up. And she said, "Hello! Would you like to see your baby girl?" And I said to myself, "A baby girl? What do you mean, a baby girl? It's surprising enough that *I* survived that, but a *baby*? A baby certainly could not have."

But she *had* survived, and the nurse brought over your mother all wrapped in pink, and the nurse said, "See? We've got her wrapped in pink."

Jaci, 2006

"Well, isn't that nice?" my mother said, sassily. "They wrapped me up in pink." She was examining the ice packs that a nurse had offered to help with swollen, tender breasts. She approved of them. She'd heard some hospitals offered raspberry Popsicles to put inside your bra, which was ridiculous. The raspberry would stain your clothes.

When Charlie woke and cried, my mother picked him up. Grandma leaned forward in her chair. "Go ahead and feed him if you like," she told me. "Your mother will tell you quick-smart if you're doing it wrong."

———

5.

Jaci, 2006

Four weeks later Colin flew back to Canada. I stood at the open front door in my pyjamas, smiling wide-eyed at the taxi driver. My feet were bare in the early morning cold, and in my arms Charlie blinked and frowned.

2006

To my dearest Jaci &
Darling Charlie,

Just a little note my darling wishing I could be there to help you on your way.

If there is anything I could do for you please let me know.

You and Charlie are welcome to stay here in the sewing room any time. And very welcome.

I feel so helpless but I do hope my thoughts will help. I'll send this care of your mother for I don't have your address. Take care and let me know anything I can do.

Lots and lots of love
And care and Blessings
From Your,
Grandma Lily
XXXXX

ABOUT THE CONTRIBUTORS

CAROLINE ADDERSON is the author of four novels (*A History of Forgetting, Sitting Practice, The Sky Is Falling, Ellen in Pieces*), two collections of short stories (*Bad Imaginings, Pleased To Meet You*), as well as many books for young readers. She is also the editor and co-contributor of a non-fiction book of essays and photographs, *Vancouver Vanishes: Narratives of Demolition and Revival*. Her work has received numerous award nominations including the *Sunday Times* EFG Private Bank Short Story Award, the International IMPAC Dublin Literary Award, two Commonwealth Writers' Prizes, the Governor General's Literary Award, the Rogers' Trust Fiction Prize, and the Scotiabank Giller Prize longlist. Winner of three BC Book Prizes and three CBC Literary Awards, Caroline was also the recipient of the 2006 Marian Engel Award for mid-career achievement. She lives in Vancouver.

PETER BEHRENS' first novel, *The Law of Dreams*, won the Governor General's Literary Award for Fiction and has been published in nine languages. The *New York Times Book Review* called his second novel, *The O'Briens*, "a major achievement" and Megan O'Grady, writing in *Vogue*, calls Behrens' latest novel, *Carry Me*, "another meditation on history and destiny... that make[s] the past feel stunningly close at hand." *Carry Me* recently won The Vine Award for Canadian Jewish Literature and Behrens was cited by the jury as "a master," with his work being described as "a novel that could be, should be, read in a hundred years." A native of Montreal, Peter Behrens held a Wallace Stegner Fellowship at Stanford University and was a Fellow of Harvard University's Radcliffe Institute for Advanced Study.

JOSEPH BOYDEN's first novel, *Three Day Road*, was selected for the *Today Show* Book Club, won the Rogers Writers' Trust Fiction Prize, the CBA Libris Fiction Book of the Year Award, and the Amazon.ca/*Books in Canada* First Novel Award, and was short-listed for the Governor General's Award for Fiction. His second novel, *Through Black Spruce*, was awarded the Scotiabank Giller Prize and named the Canadian Booksellers Association Fiction Book of the Year; it also earned him the CBA's Author of the Year Award. His most recent novel, *The Orenda*, won Canada Reads and was nominated for the Scotiabank Giller Prize and the Governor General's Award for Fiction. Boyden divides his time between Northern Ontario and Louisiana.

JOAN CLARK is the author of the novels *An Audience of Chairs*, *Latitudes of Melt*, *The Victory of Geraldine Gull*, and *Eiriksdottir* as well as two story collections, three picture books, and six award-winning novels for young adults. She is the only Canadian writer to have won both the Marian Engel Award in recognition of her body of work in adult fiction and the Vicky Metcalf Award in recognition of her body of work in children's literature. Her seventh novel for young people will be published by Doubleday in 2009. Born and raised in Nova Scotia, she has lived in various places across Canada with her geotechnical engineer husband

Jack. While living in Calgary, she became a founding member of the Alberta Writers Guild and co-founded the acclaimed literary journal *Dandelion*. She now lives in St. John's, Newfoundland.

LYNN COADY is a novelist and essayist whose fiction has been garnering acclaim since her first novel, *Strange Heaven*, was published and subsequently nominated for the Governor General's Award for Fiction when she was twenty-eight. Her short story collection *Hellgoing* won the 2013 Scotiabank Giller Prize, Canada's most prestigious literary award, for which her novel *The Antagonist* was also nominated in 2011. Her books have been published in the U.K., U.S., Holland, France, and Germany. Coady has been a journalist, magazine editor, and advice columnist, and is currently writing for television. She divides her time between Edmonton and Toronto.

CHRISTY ANN CONLIN is the author of *The Memento* and *Heave*, which was a *Globe and Mail* "Top 100" book, a finalist for the Amazon.ca First Novel Award, the Thomas H. Raddall Atlantic Fiction Award, and the Dartmouth Book Award, and longlisted for CBC's Canada Reads in 2011. She is also the author of a young adult novel, *Dead Time*. Conlin was the pet columnist at the *Globe and Mail* and hosted the 2012 CBC summer radio series *Fear Itself*. Her short fiction, essays, reviews, and photos have appeared in numerous publications, including *Brick*, *Best Canadian Stories*, *Geist*, *Numéro Cinq*, the *Globe and Mail*, *Room Magazine*, *Chatelaine* and *Canadian Geographic*. Conlin studied creative writing at the University of British Columbia, where she received the William Rhea Fellowship in Television Writing. She lives in the Annapolis Valley, Nova Scotia.

KAREN CONNELLY is the author of the national bestseller *The Lizard Cage*, which won the prestigious Orange Prize for New Writers, and was shortlisted for both the Kiriyama Prize and the International IMPAC Dublin Literary Award. Connelly's first book of poetry, *The Small Words in My Body*, won the Pat Lowther Award. Her first book of prose, *Touch the Dragon: A Thai Journal* — an account of the year she spent in Thailand at seventeen — won the Governor General's Literary Award for Nonfiction in 1993; at twenty-four, she was the youngest writer ever to win that prize. She is currently working on a memoir set in the refugee camps and among the rebel armies along the Burmese-Thai border. She lives in Toronto, Ontario.

AFUA COOPER is an established writer of nonfiction, history, and poetry. Her book, *The Hanging of Angélique*, was a finalist for the Governor General's Literary Award for Nonfiction. She is co-author of *We're Rooted Here and They Can't Pull Us Up: Essays in African-Canadian Women's History*, which won the prestigious Joseph Brant Award, and has published five volumes of poetry, including the acclaimed *Copper Women and Other Poems*. She has a Ph.D. in African-Canadian history with specialties in slavery and abolition. She now holds the Ruth Wynn Woodward Chair in Women's Studies at Simon Fraser University, Burnaby, British Columbia.

ANNE FLEMING is the author of five books: *Pool-Hopping and Other Stories*, *Anomaly*, *Gay Dwarves of America*, all fiction; *poemw*, a book of poems; and *The Goat*, a novel for children. Her books have been nominated for many nice awards.

BILL GASTON is the author of several collections of fiction, including the Scotiabank Giller Prize finalist *Mount Appetite*, the Governor General's Award finalists *Gargoyles* and *Juliet Was a Surprise*, as well as the acclaimed novels *Sointula*, *The Good Body*, and most recently *The World*. His work appears in *Granta*, *Tin House*, and *Best Canadian Stories*, and has been translated into several languages. Gaston was the inaugural recipient of the Writers' Trust of Canada Timothy Findley Award, for a distinguished body of work. He lives in Victoria, British Columbia, with his wife, author Dede Crane, and their four children.

CURTIS GILLESPIE is the critically acclaimed author of the novel *Crown Shyness* and the memoir *Playing Through*. He has received numerous awards for his fiction, including the Danuta Gleed Award. His nonfiction has appeared in publications in Canada, the United States, and Britain, and has earned him three National Magazine Awards. He lives in Edmonton, Alberta, with his wife and two daughters.

PAULINE HOLDSTOCK is the author of five novels, one story collection, and a collection of essays. She has been nominated for the Amazon.ca First Novel Award, the CBC Literary Award, the Commonwealth Writers' Prize, and the Scotiabank Giller Prize. She has won the Matrix/Random House Prize, the Federation of B.C. Writers Prize for Fiction, the Prairie Fire Personal Journalism Prize, and the Ethel Wilson Fiction Prize. Her work has been published in Canada, the U.K., and the U.S. Originally from England, she now lives in Vancouver Island, British Columbia.

MARTIN LEVIN is the co-author of an unstaged play about the world's worst film director, and a contributor to the anthology of essays by men, *What I Meant to Say*. He lives in Toronto, Ontario.

SANDRA MARTIN is an award-winning writer and journalist. Her most recent book is the bestseller *A Good Death: Making the Most of Our Final Choices*, which won the B.C. National Award for Canadian Non-fiction and was a finalist for both the Donner Prize in Public Policy and the J.W. Dafoe Book Prize. Her other books include *Great Canadian Lives: A Cultural History of Modern Canada through the Art of the Obit*, and *The First Man in My Life: Daughters Write about Their Fathers*. Born and educated in Montreal, Quebec, Martin lives in Toronto, Ontario, with her husband, Roger Hall. She has two adult children and three grandchildren.

LEAH MCLAREN is a columnist and novelist. In 2013, she won a gold National Magazine Award in the arts feature category for her work in *Toronto Life* magazine. She is the bestselling author of *The Continuity Girl* and *A Better Man*. She was born in rural Ontario, grew up in a small town, and now splits her time between Toronto and London, England, where she shares a home with her husband and two boys.

JACLYN MORIARTY is the critically acclaimed author of the young adult novels *Feeling Sorry for Celia*, *The Year of Secret Assignments*, and most recently the *Colours of Madeleine* trilogy. She is also the author of the upcoming middle-grade fiction, *The Extremely Inconvenient Adventures of Bronte Mettlestone* (Fall, 2018). Born in Australia, Moriarty lived in Canada for several years and now makes her home in Sydney, Australia.

STEPHANIE NOLEN is the *Globe and Mail*'s Africa correspondent. She is a three-time winner of both the National Newspaper Award and the Amnesty International Award for Human Rights Reporting. She is also the author of *Shakespeare's Face, Promised the Moon: The Untold Story of the First Women in the Space Race*, and the bestselling *28: Stories of AIDS in Africa*, which was nominated for the Governor General's Literary Award for Nonfiction. She lives in Johannesburg, South Africa, with her partner and son.

KATHY PAGE is the author of six novels, including *The Story of My Face*, which was longlisted for the Orange Prize, and *Alphabet*, which was a Governor General's Literary Award finalist. She has written short fiction and script for radio and TV. "The Second Spring after Liberation," which appears in her story collection *As In Music*, won the Bridport Prize. She has taught writing at universities and other institutions in the U.K., Finland, Estonia, and Canada. She lives with her husband and two children in Salt Spring Island, British Columbia.

CHRISTINE POUNTNEY is the acclaimed author of the novels *Sweet Jesus, Last Chance Texaco*, which was longlisted for the Orange Prize, and *The Best Way You Know How*. Born in Vancouver, British Columbia, she grew up in Montreal, Quebec, and lived for six years in London, England. She now lives in Toronto, Ontario.

EDEET RAVEL is the author of *Ten Thousand Lovers*, which was translated into several languages and received many literary distinctions including a nomination for the Governor General's Award. Her novel *Look For Me* won the Hugh MacLennan Prize, and *A Wall of Light* was a finalist for the Scotiabank Giller Prize, the Regional Commonwealth Prize, and won the Jewish Book Award of Canada and the I. J. Segal Award. Edeet's writing for young readers has garnered numerous honours; her most recent Young Adult novel, *Held*, has been nominated for the CLA Young Adult Book of the Year, the Saskatchewan Willow Award, the Pennsylvania School Librarians Association Top Forty, and the Arthur Ellis Crime Award. Her Young Adult novel *The Saver* has been adapted for film by Wiebke von Carolsfeld. The film has received awards around the globe. Edeet holds a Ph.D. in Jewish Studies from McGill University and now lives in Guelph, Ontario. Her name is pronounced ee-DEET.

MICHAEL REDHILL was born in Baltimore, Maryland in 1966, but has lived in Toronto most of his life. He is a novelist, playwright, and poet. Educated in the United States and Canada, he took seven years to complete a three-year B.A. in acting, film, and finally, English. Since 1988, he has published sixteen books, including five collections of poetry and eight works of fiction. He has been the publisher and one of the editors of *Brick*, a journal of things literary since 1998. His first novel, *Martin Sloane*, was nominated for the Scotiabank Giller Prize and won the *Books in Canada* / Amazon.ca Best First Novel Prize. His second novel, *Consolation*, won the City of Toronto Book Award and was long-listed for the Man Booker Prize. His poetry includes *Light-crossing* and *Lake Nora Arms*, and his play *Building Jerusalem* won a Dora for Best New Play and a Chalmers Award for Playwriting. In 2012, he revealed he is the author of the crime books of Inger Ash Wolfe. His most recent literary novel, *Bellevue Square*, won the Scotiabank Giller Prize. He has two sons and lives in Toronto.

ESTA SPALDING is at the forefront of a new generation of Canadian poets. Her first book, *Carrying Place*, was nominated for the Gerald R. Lampert Award and her second, *Anchoress*, was a finalist for the CBA Libris Award. Her third book, *Lost August*, won the Pat Lowther Memorial Award and her fourth book, *The Wife's Account*, was nominated for it. She is an award-winning film and television writer and the co-author of a novel, *Mere*. She lives in Vancouver, British Columbia.

EMILY URQUHART is a journalist with a doctorate in folklore and draws on both backgrounds in her writing. Her work has appeared in *Azure*, the *Globe and Mail*, *Hakai Magazine*, and the *Walrus*, and in 2014 she won a National Magazine Award. Her first book, *Beyond the Pale: Folklore, Family, and the Mystery of Our Hidden Genes,* was a *Globe and Mail* Best Book of 2015 and was shortlisted for the B.C. National Award for Canadian Non-Fiction, the Kobo Emerging Writer Prize, and the B.C. Book Prize for non-fiction. She lives in Kitchener, Ontario, with her husband and their two young children.

CLAIRE WILKSHIRE is a freelance editor and writer. She was a founding member of the fiction collective The Burning Rock, and her stories have been published alongside Lisa Moore's, Michael Winter's, and Ramona Dearing's in the Burning Rock anthologies *Hearts Larry Broke* and *Extremities*. She has published in *The Fiddlehead*, *Event*, *The New Quarterly*, and *Grain*. She is also co-editor, with John Metcalf, of the anthology *Writers Talking*. She holds a Ph.D. in English literature from the University of British Columbia. She lives in St. John's, Newfoundland.

ACKNOWLEDGEMENTS

WE HAD A LOT of help with the birth of this book. Thank you hugely to Lynn Henry. She is unerring and generous and ultra-smart, a great editor and friend. Thank you also to Janie Yoon for her dedication, wise advice, and lassoing capabilities.

Thank you to the whole team at Anansi. We feel lucky to be in such strong hands. Thank you to Sarah MacLachlan, Matt Williams, Laura Repas, and Julie Wilson.

The first edition of our book had a beautiful cover design for which we are grateful to Bill Douglas.

The contributors wrote with great honesty, and we thank them for their generosity.

Lastly and lovingly, we thank Steve Crocker and Bill Gaston for just about everything.

ABOUT THE EDITORS

DEDE CRANE is the critically acclaimed author of the novels *Sympathy* and *Every Happy Family*, a collection of stories *The Cult of Quick Repair*, and two novels for teens. Shortlisted for the CBC Literary Awards, a CLA Award, the Butler Book Prize among others, she lives in British Columbia, with her husband, writer Bill Gaston.

LISA MOORE is the acclaimed author of *Caught, February,* and *Alligator. Caught* was a finalist for the Rogers Writers' Trust Fiction Prize and the Scotiabank Giller Prize. *February* won CBC's Canada Reads competition, was longlisted for the Man Booker Prize, and was named a *New Yorker* Best Book of the Year, and a *Globe and Mail* Top 100 Book. *Alligator* was a finalist for the Scotiabank Giller Prize, won the Commonwealth Writers' Prize (Canada and the Caribbean), and was a national bestseller. Her story collection *Open* was a finalist for the Scotiabank Giller Prize and a national bestseller. She lives in St. John's, Newfoundland.

A LIST

The A List